Profitable Sheep and Goat Farming

The Author

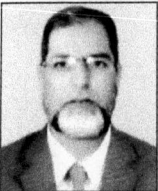

Dr. Zahoor A. Pampori graduated in Veterinary Sciences from Ranchi Veterinary College, Ranchi and has completed Ph.D degree in Animal Physiology from ICAR-National Dairy Research Institute (NDRI) Karnal, Haryana. He has served J&K State Animal Husbandry Department for 13 years in the capacity of Veterinary Assistant Surgeon and Research Officer. He got appointed as Assistant Professor in SKUAST-Kashmir and subsequently elevated as Senior Scientist. Presently, Dr. Pampori is posted as Senior Scientist cum Incharge, Mountain Research Centre for Sheep & Goat, SKUAST-K, Shuhama. He has published more than 30 research papers in journals of repute, two manuals and a book entitled "Field-cum-Laboratory Procedures in Animal Health Care" from Daya Publishing House, New Delhi.

Profitable Sheep and Goat Farming

– Author –

Zahoor A. Pampori

FACULTY OF VETERINARY SCIENCES AND ANIMAL HUSBANDRY,
SKUAST-K, SHUHAMA,
ALUSTENG, SRINAGAR- 190006
J&K

2017

Daya Publishing House®

A Division of

Astral International Pvt. Ltd.

New Delhi – 110 002

ISBN 9789386071965 (International Edition)

Published by   : **Daya Publishing House®**
                                 A Division of
                                 Astral International Pvt. Ltd.
                                 – ISO 9001:2015 Certi ied Company –
                                 4736/23, Ansari Road, Darya Ganj
                                 New Delhi-110 002
                                 Ph. 011-43549197, 23278134
                                 E-mail: info@astralint.com
                                 Website: www.astralint.com

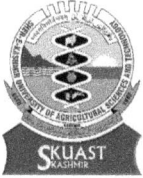

Sher-e-Kashmir
University of Agricultural Sciences & Technology (Kashmir)
Shalimar, Srinagar. (Jammu & Kashmir)

Prof (Dr) M. T. Banday
M.V.Sc; PhD; Fellow National
Associate Director Extension
(Animal Science)

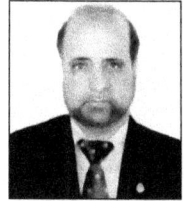

Foreword

The rapidly changing pattern of demand for livestock and livestock products are a great challenge nowadays. Most of the population of India are residing in the rural areas and depend on agriculture and animal husbandry for their sustainability. Sheep and goat husbandry in India is an age old business where the real stake holders of genetic diversity of sheep and goat have been the poor farmers. Both these livestock also play an important role in fulfillment of nutrient requirement of the family and also generate employment. The extent to which the rural poor will be benefited from them depends on how livestock can be integrated into developing market and whether the products from them benefit the rural poor as consumers as well as producers. Their significance which is now being exploited in several countries is that they are small livestock in high demand and can thrive well on low inputs and local resources. The potential challenges of this sector has many shortfalls such as low availability of quality germplasm/quality feed resources/ poor processing and value addition infrastructure/ poor health delivery system, failure in exploiting the potential of indigenous breeds.

In view of this a book entitled "**Profitable Sheep and Goat Farming**" has been written. The book deals with scientific production and management of sheep and goats. All the important topics related to these two species have been covered in detail and which are well planned/explained using simple language with sketches/ illustrations and tables wherever necessary. The book contains updated information as per revised VCI curriculum presented in 15 chapters for undergraduate students of Bachelor of Veterinary Sciences & Animal Husbandry in, post-graduate and PhD scholars from LPM/APM discipline in the various State Agricultural/Veterinary universities of the country. It will also help the interested students for preparation of competitive examination both in public and private sector. I hope that all concerned with livestock sector will find the information in this book useful.

I appreciate the author for taking the initiative to write this book.

M.T BANDAY

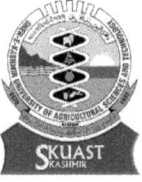

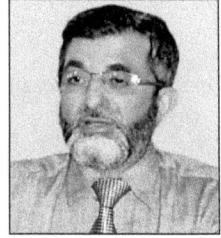

Prof (Dr) Sarfaraz. A. Wani
MvSc.Ph.D.,
Dean

Message from Dean's Desk

Livestock is the most important component of Indian agriculture sector that contributes about 4.1 per cent to the national GDP and 28 per cent to the agricultural GDP. Crop agriculture has become more vulnerable to the changing climatic conditions whereas animal agriculture is more stable, more sustainable and less vulnerable to changing climate, thus a promising source of sustained livelihood and food security. Livestock also serves as an insurance substitute, especially for poor rural households during draughts, floods or natural calamities that can easily be sold for subsistence. Sheep and goat farming is an age old endeavour of millions of small holders of rural India which is highly gender sensitive. over 90 percent of activities related to care and management of livestock, is carried out by family's women folk. The small holders produce milk, meat, fibre, skin etc for the community with virtually no capital, resource and formal training. Sheep and goat farming is a proficient practice that can create new employment opportunities for the unemployed educated youth. Therefore, structuring and editing a book on "Profitable sheep and goat farming" by Dr. Zahoor A Pampori is most welcome and need of the day. The book has comprehensive coverage on almost every feature of farming including housing, nutrition, handling, disease control, fodder and manure management as well as care in various phases of growth and production in sheep and goat.

I am sure that this book will be of immense value and beneficial to the farmers engaged in small ruminant farming, interesting entrepreneurs, academicians as well as students of animal science.

Prof. Dr. Sarfaraz A Wani

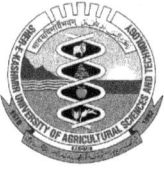

Sher-e-Kashmir University of Agricultural Sciences & Technology of Kashmir

Prof. (Dr.) Nazeer Ahmed
Vice-Chancellor
FISVS, FHSI, FISHRD & FCHAI

www.skuastkashmir.ac.in

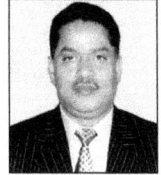

Message from Vice-Chancellor

Sheep and goats are the most affordable animals in the world which have adopted in different climatic conditions. These small ruminants can be projected as future animal in contemporary changing climatic scenario owing to their higher survival rates under harsh conditions and significant water economy as compared to cattle. Sheep and goats are relatively cheap and are easily acquired through purchase or customary means by familied recovering from a catastrophe such as drought, floods, storms or war which subsequently becomes a valuable asset, providing milk meat and financial security to the family. Sheep and goat husbandry in India is essentially an endeavour of millions of small holders who rear animals on "crop residues" and "common property resources", which constitutes an indispensable source of their livelihood. India stands first in goat population and second in sheep in the world, with 135.17 million goat and 65.07 million sheep respectively. Further, about 90 per cent of women folk are associated with the rearing of animals including sheep & goats thus serving as an important sector for women empowerment. The increasing demand for food products of animal origin due to swelling population, increasing income and urbanization has lead to small ruminant enterprise for meeting intended demands.

Acknowledging the importance of sheep and goats in the national economy and nutritional security, sheep farming is one of the most important sector in agriculture industry to invest in, therefore, any effort to upkeep sheep & goat farming is quite appreciating. From the contents of the book it is perceived that the author has made a noble attempt to assemble all facets of farming practices related to sheep and goats, in this comprehensive handout, to disseminate the husbandry knowledge to its stakeholders. It is hoped that this book proves beneficial to livestock farmers, veterinarians, academicians as well as students of animal science. I take this opportunity to congratulate the author who is our faculty member and wish him a great success.

Prof. (Dr.) Nazeer Ahmed

Shalimar Srinagar-190025, J&K, India
Phone: (O) 0194-2462159, 2464028 Fax: 0194-2462160 (R) 0194-2463655, 2436700 Fax: 0194-2461543
E-mail: vc@skuastkashmir.ac.in, skuastkvc@gmail.com

Preface

Livestock farming has remained an important integral component of Indian agriculture fanning system, that contributes in many folds, on one hand it provides food and nutritional security through different nutrient rich animal products like milk, meat and eggs and on the other hand, contributes to national economy and generates employment. Livestock is considered a bank on four legs and serves as cash in hand with the farmer. In present changing agro-climatic scenario with unpredicted, unprecedented weather events, livestock gives a cushing effect against the crop failures because animal agriculture is more stable, more sustainable, more promising and less vulnerable to changing climate. Furthermore, livestock are closely linked to the social and cultural lives of several million resource-poor farmers, for whom animal ownership ensures varying degrees of sustainable farming and economic stability. The history of domestication of sheep and goats goes back to Neolithic era between 11000 and 9000 BC.

India stands 1st in goat population and 2nd in sheep population in the world, with 135.17 million goats and 65.07 million sheep as per the ^9tl' livestock census which constitutes 16.1 per cent and 6.4 per cent of world goat and sheep population respectively. In the year 2012-13 goat contributed 16 per cent and sheep 7 per cent to the total meat production of 5.9 million tonnes and further sheep produced 46.1 million kg wool during the said year. The availability of meat in India is only about 15g/person/day against the ICMR-recommendation of 30g/person/day. Similarly, in developing countries, annual meat consumption is expected to increase from 36.4 kg in 1999 to 45.30 kg in 2030. In India, there is significant dearth of the meat when equated with the-ICMR recommendations or world average meat consumption. All these trends in meat demand and production warrants technology solutions in livestock production systems. Over the time livestock farming has witnessed huge changes in its husbandry. Animals are now being provided with nutritious food, shelter, better health care and bred selectively for more yield and quality product. Sheep and goats have served poor people's most reliable livelihood resource since their domestication during Neolithic Revolution. Worldwide over 100 million people in arid areas, have only possible source of livelihood by grazing small ruminants. Grazing sheep and goats can improve soil and vegetation cover and plant and animal biodiversity. Sheep and goats thrive well in varied climatic conditions, get adapted easily to environment, require less care and management and are suitable for meat, milk, wool, skins and manure production. Mutton and Chowan is consumed throughout the country without involving any religious taboo.

Together, the goat and sheep rearing households constitute 15 per cent of the total number of households in the country. Acknowledging the wide distribution of small ruminants among the marginal and small farmers of rural India, owing to their tremendous sustaining potential in changing agro-climatic conditions, they have to be projected as the 'Future Animals' for rural and urban prosperity. There is a strong driving force in the form of expanding human population, urbanization, improved income and higher demands for food of animal origin that will definitely encourage the farmers and educated unemployed youth to invest in the small ruminant livestock sector in coming years. As an incharge of Mountain Research Centre for Sheep and Goat, SKUAST-Kashmir, I often receive many marginal/small farmers as well as educated unemployed youth interested in fanning, asking for guidelines in small ruminant farming, this stimulated me to get equipped with a documented package to guide interested ones about the care and management of sheep and goats. Initially I framed a year calendar for management of sheep and goats that was supportive to the farmers in general, but was not serving the needs of all stakeholders in a comprehensive way. All these facts, infact, instigated me to come-up with a comprehensive digest containing necessary package of farming practices for small ruminants to help livestock farmers, entrepreneurs and all other stakeholders including veterinarians and paravets in keeping and managing the animals properly for subsistence and profitability. The book contains a package of farm practices encompassing housing, handling, feeding, health care, record keeping, fodder and manure management as well as project reporting for sheep and goats. This precise package of practices hopefully shall benefit all the farmers engaged in small ruminant farming as well as all those educated entrepreneurs that are willing to take livestock rearing as their carrier option. It will guide through all aspects of sheep and goat farm management. I wish this book help farmers in managing their livestock and teachers equally in imparting academic instructions to veterinary graduates. I would like to acknowledge and appreciate Astral Publications (P) Ltd. who came in way to help me in disseminating the package of practices from their desk to the interested ones all over the globe.

Zahoor A Pampori

Contents

Chapter 1

Importance of Livestock Farming in Livelihood and Food Security

Livestock farming is the rearing of animals for food or pleasure or for other human uses. Animal rearing has its origin in the transition of cultures to settled farming communities from hunter-gatherer's lifestyle. The word 'Livestock' applies primarily to cattle or dairy cows, buffalo, sheep, goats, pigs, horses and chickens. Today, even animals like donkeys, mules, rabbits, turkeys, ducks, geese, guinea fowl and insects such as bees are being raised as part of livestock farming. Mankind has been utilizing different animal species from the dawn of civilization for a variety of purposes *viz.* production of milk, meat, wool, egg and leather. Apart from these, various animal species are also used for draught power, companionship, entertainment, research experimentation, sports, security *etc.* Livestock farming has historically been a backbone of national economy while providing livelihood, food security, prosperity and employment generation.

Livestock, particularly the ruminants, thrive on pasture forage, harvested roughage, or by-product feeds, as well as non-protein nitrogen such as urea and convert them into nutrient rich meat, milk and wool for human use. The skins or hides and even hair of these animals have been used to make blankets, clothing, shoes and the like. The hoofs and horns of these farm animals have been used to make items like buttons and combs. Even the animal-wastes do not go waste rather make an excellent natural fertilizer. Livestock is considered a bank on four legs and serves as cash in hand with the farmer. In rural India it is offered as dowry with a bride.

The livestock sector has emerged as one of the key components of agricultural growth in developing countries in the recent years. The main activity of rural populace has remained green agriculture for long past but present changing climate scenario with unpredicted, unprecedented extreme weather events has made the crops more vulnerable to losses and thus threatening the economic stability. In contrast animal agriculture is more stable, more sustainable, more promising and less vulnerable to changing climate, thus a strong hope for sustained livelihood and food security.

The Indian livestock farming is the endeavor of small holders and it is a centuries old tradition. Over 70 percentage of the rural households in India depend on livestock farming for supplementary income. The sector is highly gender sensitive and over 90 percent of activities related to care and management of livestock, is carried out by family's women folk, and thus serves a strong sector for women empowerment. The livestock sector employs eight percent of the country's labour force, including many small and marginal farmers, women and landless agricultural workers. Although contribution of livestock towards Gross Domestic Product at national level has reduced but still it is considered strong pillar of Indian economy and around 27.25 per cent of agriculture GDP is contributed by livestock sector that highlights the importance of livestock farming in national economy. As per 19th Livestock census, 2012 (GOI, 2014) India's livestock sector is one of the largest in the world with a holding of 11.6 per cent of world livestock population which consists sheep (7.14 per cent) and goats (17.93). India has huge livestock population of 512 million which mainly includes cattle, buffaloes, goats, sheep and pigs. Contribution of sheep and goats in total livestock population is 12.71 and 26.4 per cent, respectively. Total meat production including poultry meat was 5.9 million tons in 2012-13 as compared to 1.9 million tons in 2001-02. Nearly 16 per cent and 7 per cent of the total production of meat is contributed by goat and sheep respectively. The availability of meat in India is only about 15g/person/day against the ICMR recommendation of 30g/person/day. In India, total wool production has increased from 27.5 million kg in 1950-51 to 46.1 million kg in 2012-13. Between 1983 and 2004, the share of animal products in the total food expenditure increased from 21.8 per cent to 25.0 per cent in urban areas and from 16.1 per cent to 21.4 per cent in rural areas. Despite deceleration, growth in livestock sector remained about 1.5 times higher than in the crop sector which implies its critical role in cushioning agricultural growth.

Livestock farming presents bright future because over the next 15 years, global demand for meat is expected to increase by 40 per cent as a result of swelling human population and their increased preference in animal protein-rich diets. World's livestock sector is growing at unprecedented rate and the driving force behind it is enormous surge in human population, rising incomes, urbanization and rise of supermarkets especially in cities and towns. Annual meat production is projected to increase to 376 million tons by 2030 in the world. Similarly, in developing countries meat consumption is expected to increase from 36.4 kg in 1999 to 45.30 kg in 2030. All these trends are encouraging in future growth of livestock sector and further small ruminant is more suitable and hardy animal to thrive best in changing agro-climatic conditions that may project sheep and goats as "Future Animals" for farming. For a growing human population, and increasing demands of animal foods, the development of livestock sector is indispensable. From livelihood perspective, livestock farming is considered as an important instrument in poverty alleviation and this sector is emerging as an important growth leverage to national economy.

Increasing trends in meat production and demand warrants technology solutions in agricultural and livestock production systems to address the demand of meat supply for an expected population. Increasing livestock horizontally will have environmental/climatic concerns and animal welfare issues that need to be addressed in coming days. Over the time livestock farming has witnessed huge changes in its husbandry. Animals are now being provided with food, shelter and bred selectively. They are given nutritious processed feed to boost normal growth and production. Selective and cross breeding programs in livestock husbandry have now given us excellent breeds of farm animals that yield more and quality product. Animal management and health care has witnessed huge change. Vaccinations and dosing in the livestock are now routine practices at farm. Outdoor farming of livestock in bigger enclosures like ranches and fenced pastures are some strategies for efficient use of available resources. Chaffing, urea treatment, molasses or fungal treatment of low quality straws have increased the nutritive values of straws and thus more returns.

Table 1: Livestock Population (millions) as per 1951, 2007 and 2012 Livestock Census in India

Sl.No.	Livestock	Livestock Census (1951)	Livestock Census (2007)	Livestock Census (2012)	Per cent Increase/ Decrease (2007-2012)
1.	Cattle	155.3	199.08	190.9	−4.1
2.	Buffaloes	43.4	105.34	108.7	3.19
	Total bovines (Cattle, Buffalo, Yak and Mithun)	198.7	304.42	299.98	−1.57
3.	Sheep	39.1	71.56	65.07	−9.07
4.	Goats	47.2	140.54	135.17	−3.82
5.	Pigs	4.4	11.13	10.29	−7.54
6.	Horses and ponies	1.5	0.61	0.62	2.12
7.	Mules	0.06	0.14	0.20	43.07
8.	Donkeys	1.3	0.44	0.32	−27.17
9.	Camels	0.6	0.52	0.40	−22.63
	Total livestock	**292.8**	**529.7**	**512**	**−3.33**

Despite having great deal of improvement in technology sector related to livestock farming, yet the livestock sector has to go a long way to harvest the real benefits of recent technologies developed in the sector. The livestock sector did not receive the policy and financial attention it deserved. The sector received only about 12 per cent of the total public expenditure on agriculture and allied sectors, which is disproportionately lesser than its contribution to agricultural GDP. The sector too has been neglected by the financial institutions. The share of livestock in the total agricultural credit has hardly ever exceeded 4 per cent in the total (short-term, medium-term and long-term). The institutional mechanisms to protect animals against risk are not strong enough. Currently, only 6 per cent of the animal heads (excluding poultry) are provided insurance cover. Livestock extension has remained grossly neglected in the past. Only about 5 per cent of the farm households in India access information on livestock technology. These indicate an apathetic outreach of the financial and information delivery systems. The extent to which the pro-poor potential of livestock can be harnessed would depend on how technology, institutions, policies and financial support address the constraints of the sector. The number-driven growth in livestock production may not sustain in the long run due to its increasing stress on the limited natural resources. The future growth has to come from improvements in technology and service delivery systems leading to accelerated productivity, processing and marketing.

Why Sheep and Goat Farming?

Having understood the importance of livestock farming and its prospects in the country as a whole, let us peep into the advantages of sheep and goat farming in our country.

☆ Traditionally, sheep and goat rearing has been the primary source of livelihood for shepherds, who often belong to distinct communities viz Raikas of Rajasthan, Dhangars of Maharashtra, Kurubas of Karnataka, Chopans and changpas of J&K. Similarly, the livelihood of Gojar and Bakerwals of northern states of Himachal, Punjab and J&K are totally reliant on sheep and goat which they rear in a migratory system of rearing.

☆ Sheep and goats are small sized animals requiring little space and housing, as such permit them to be maintained on a limited area. Therefore, sheep and goat farming is largely with marginal and small farmers of the country. In rural India, where over 15-20 per cent families are landless and about 80 per cent of the land holders belong to the category of small and marginal farmers, prefer to own sheep and goat, that infact play a very vital role in their livelihood security.

☆ Sheep and goat husbandry in India is essentially an endeavor of millions of small holders who rear animals on "Crop Residues" and "Common Property Resources". The small holders produce milk, meat, fiber, skin etc for the community with virtually no capital, resource and formal training. The total number of households and household enterprises, both rural and urban, which rear/own sheep and goats are 4.55 and 33.01 million respectively. Together, the goat and sheep rearing households constitute 15 per cent of the total number of households in the country. Similarly, non-household enterprises and institutions which rear/own sheep and goats are 8,010 and 25,189 respectively.

☆ They are hardy, disease resistant and widely adapted. They thrive well and reproduce well in tropical, cold, humid as well as dry regions.

☆ They are gentle and easy to control. Their small size makes them suitable for backyard slaughter and the meat can be consumed by the family.

☆ The breeding animals are inexpensive. The capital investment for starting the farming of small ruminants is far less as compared to farming of large animals and returns of investment are within a very short period.

✮ They are close grazers and browsers hence consume a wide variety of grasses, weeds, forbs, bushes, shrubs, tree leaves and crop residues that would otherwise go waste and cause pollution. Sheep because of its close grazing behavour is believed a good weed destroyer.

✮ They are efficient converters of the sparse vegetation available in wastelands, community grazing lands of arid, semiarid and mountainous regions into milk, meat, skin, fibre and manure while utilizing traditional and under employed manpower.

✮ Goat meat (chevon) and sheep meat (mutton) is preferred over other meats because it is leaner and there are no religious taboos against its consumption.

✮ The vast population and large genetic resource available in the country are the strengths of the sector.

✮ They are mostly looked after by the women in the family and hence offers an opportunity for empowerment of women through small ruminant-based livelihood improvement.

✮ Sheep and goat are efficient reproducers and on an average a female can give birth to 1-2 kids/lambs per delivery.

✮ Commercial sheep and or goat farming business can create new employment opportunity for the unemployed educated youth. Easy bank loan for farming business is available in the country. Several centrally sponsored schemes are operational in the States for sheep and goat rearing.

✮ There are numerous recognized sheep and goat breeds in our country which are famous for meat, milk and fiber. Many exotic breeds famous for meat and milk are also well adapted in different pockets of the country.

Chapter 2

Housing of Sheep and Goats

Sheep and goat do not require any special housing or concrete building rather fencing in open fields, thatched roof sheds usually do suffice. However, in temperate regions the livestock mostly remain indoor during winter, therefore require proper housing or shelter to combat chilling cold and at the same time keep healthy. Further the changing climate with extreme weather events has posed demand for animal shelter in subtropics too. Good, comfortable and appropriate housing for sheep and goat is very important. It keeps the animal free from all types of adverse vagaries of weather besides facilitate feeding and watering in a hygienic manner. Provision of simple shed with low cost housing material is enough for sheep and goat for its optimum production efficiency.When the animals are taken for grazing during the day time and sheltered only during night, the covered space will be enough in tropics. However, when the animals are housed intensively as in winter in Kashmir, the pen and run system of housing is suitable.

While constructing shelter for sheep and goat following points must be kept in consideration for animal comfort and successful farming business.

☆ The animal house should be constructed away from the cities preferably in rural areas or in foot hills where enough grazing land will be available.

☆ Soil must be suitable for strong foundation. Marshy, clay, sandy, rock soils are not suitable but loamy and gravely soils are best suited for building construction.

☆ The location should have road connectivity, clean water supply, electricity and market availability.

☆ The house/shed should be constructed in an elevated area to prevent water lodging and stagnation.

☆ It should be having east-west orientation with generous provision for ventilation/air movement to dry the floor and sunlight for most of the day.

☆ Sheds with mud floor are suitable but brick floor with sloop on one side is preferred in our given climatic conditions.

☆ Floors of the shed should be firm, easily cleanable and having the capacity to absorb water. Proper drainage is must.

☆ Elevated floors of wooden batons with gaps in between are preferable to separate excreta and keep floor dry and clean.

☆ In the case of wooden-batten flooring, the width of each baton should vary from 7.5 to 10.0 cm and the thickness between 2.5 cm and 4.0 cm. The sides of the planks should be well rounded and the clearance between two planks shall range between 1.0 cm and 1.5 cm to facilitate the disposal of dung and urine.

☆ The wooden-batten flooring shall be constructed at a height of at least one metre above the ground level.

☆ Walls of the shed should be free from cracks or holes. It should be such that can easily be cleaned and disinfected.

☆ Roofs should be constructed of cost effective material like thatch, cardboard/plywood, asbestos roofing. However, in temperate Kashmir valley you need to have second roofing of galvanized iron sheets to resist rain and snow during harsh winter. Gable roofing is generally preferred.

☆ There is no restriction for the length of the shelter, however breadth of shed should not exceed 12 meter and optimum breadth of shelter is 8 meter.

☆ The long shed can be partitioned lengthwise to form equal compartments for effective management.

☆ Height of the roof at animal should be 2.5 meter and height at ridge should be 3.5 meter.

☆ The height of chain link used for open space should be 4 feet. The length of the overhang should be 75cm – 1 meter.

☆ Clean drinking water and electric power supply should be available for animals.

☆ Fodder trees can be grown around the shed, which acts as a source of fodder for the growing goats.

☆ Housing should be nearer to the grazing fields.

☆ Shed should be having manger for feed and fodder at a recommended density.

☆ Water troughs should be placed in the runs rather than inside the sheds.

☆ The manger may be either of cement concrete or of wood with two compartments for providing feed and hay.

☆ A separate hay rack may also be provided by fixing it at level or slightly below the heads of the animals.

☆ With the help of clamps, the manger may be raised within the height ranging between 45 and 60cm from the ground.

☆ The water trough may be of cement concrete or galvanized steel pails or buckets and may be fixed or hanging from a hook fixed to the walls.

☆ The manger may also be of portable type. The number of mangers and water troughs in each shed may vary according to the number of animals.

☆ Every house/shed should have a foot bath at its entrance. The foot bath may be of galvanized iron sheet or of brick in cement mortar embedded in the soil at the entrance of shed. It should always have antiseptic like phenyl, PP solution or chlorhexadine in it to restrict foot infections and spread of other contaminants.

The space requirement for sheep and goat is as follows for consideration while raising shelter for them.

Age Groups	Covered Space (sq.m)	Open Space (sq.m)
Up to 3 months	0.2-0.25	0.4-0.5
3 months to 6 months	0.5-0.75	1.0-1.5
6 months to 12 months	0.75-1.0	1.5-2.0
Adult animal	1.5	3.0
Male, Pregnant or lactating ewe/doe	1.5-2.0	3.0- 4.0

Floor space requirement per animal (BIS standard)

Types of Animals	Minimum Floor Space per Animal (sq.m)
Ram or buck in groups	1.8
Ram or buck - individual	3.2
Lambs or kids - in group	0.4
Weaner in groups	0.8
yearling or goatlings	0.9
Ewe or doe in groups	1.0
Ewe with lamb	1.5

Feeding and watering space requirement

Type of Animal	Space per Animal (cm)	Width of Manger/ Water Trough (cm)	Depth of Manger/ Water Trough (cm)	Height of Inner Wall of Manger/ Water Trough (cm)
Sheep and goat	40–50	50	30	35
Kid/lamb	30–35	50	20	25

While taking sheep and goat rearing as a commercial enterprise, the organized farm should have following different sheds/rooms.

1. General flock shed (Ewe/Doe shed)
2. Ram or buck shed
3. Lambing or kidding shed
4. Lamb or kid shed
5. Sick animal shed
6. Dispensary room
7. Shearing and store room
8. Attendant's room
9. Hay shed
10. Dipping tank
11. Manure pit/vermicomposting pit
12. Silage pit if possible

General Flock Shed (Ewe/Doe Shed)

☆ The flock shed is used for housing ewes or does for breeding purpose (breeding flock)

☆ The sheds should be in west-east or south –east direction and constructed in accordance to above referred specifications/guidelines.

☆ The long bigger sheds can be divided into stalls of reasonable dimension by raising partitions of wood planks or chain-link and house the animals in each stall as per the required space. The partition should not be more than one meter high from the floor.

☆ In low lying and heavy rainfall areas, the floors should preferably be elevated. Elevated flooring is preferred as it keeps animal clean and away from soiling, thereby reducing infections and favouring growth.

☆ The walls can be of bricks or hollow concrete blocks with cement or mud plaster.

☆ Proper number of windows 1.5 meter above floor to allow sunlight in and provide good ventilation should be there. Windows should be wire net covered for ventilation and safety. Roof top ventilation may also be provided in big sheds.

☆ Sufficient feeding troughs or hay racks should be placed in the sheds as per requirement.

☆ The shed should have sufficient illumination.

Ram/Buck Shed

☆ Rams or bucks for breeding purpose are housed separately in these sheds. Alternatively, wooden partitions can be raised in bigger shed to partition into stalls.

☆ The shed should be partitioned lengthwise to form equal compartments for easy management.

Lambing/Kidding Shed

☆ These sheds are being used as maternity rooms for pregnant ewe or does.

☆ The shed should have manger for holding feed and hay and a bucket for keeping water.

☆ These sheds must be clean enough in all respects to guarantee safe delivery of kids or lambs. It should have sufficient illumination.

☆ Bedding of soft material should be provided and that should be replaced frequently to ensure dry and clean flooring.

☆ The sheds should be provided with some warming devices, like room heater, infrared bulbs fixed in maternity pens, so that newborns are protected from hypothermia particularly in temperate regions of the country.

☆ The sheds may also have wooden incubators for use in emergency.

☆ The shed should be associated with the main flock shed for easy operations during lambing or kidding.

Lamb/Kid Shed

☆ Lambs or kids from weaning up to attaining maturity are housed separately in these sheds.

☆ By making suitable partitions in a larger shed, unweaned, weaned but immature and nearby maturity lambs can be housed separately.

☆ On larger farms, however, three separate sheds may be constructed to house three categories of kids or lambs.

☆ The shed shall be partitioned breadth wise dividing into two compartments.

☆ Sheds should be provided with manger facilities for rations/concentrates and fodder.

Sick Animal Shed

☆ There must be a sick animal shed for segregating ailing and disabled animals in organized farms.

☆ The sheds are necessary to take good care of ailing stock and keep healthy ones away from sick for safety.

☆ Sick animal sheds may be constructed away from the other sheds. These sheds may be small to house only few animals at a time.

☆ The lower half of the door may be made of wooden planks and the upper half of wire-netting and similarly windows with a wire net covering to have proper, safe ventilation in the shed.

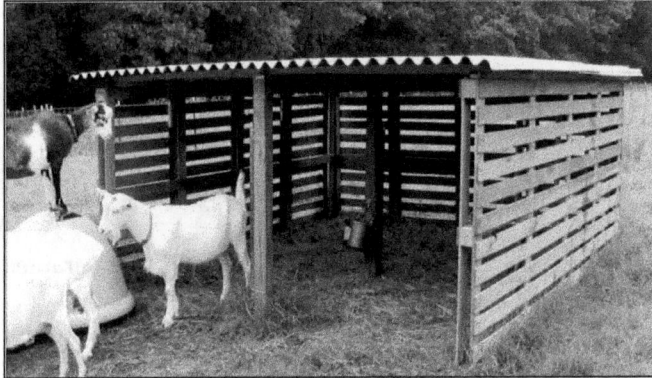

Low Cost House.

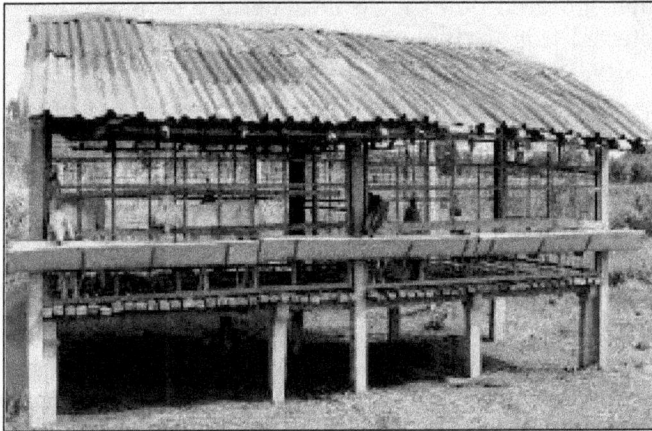

Shed with Elevated Floor.

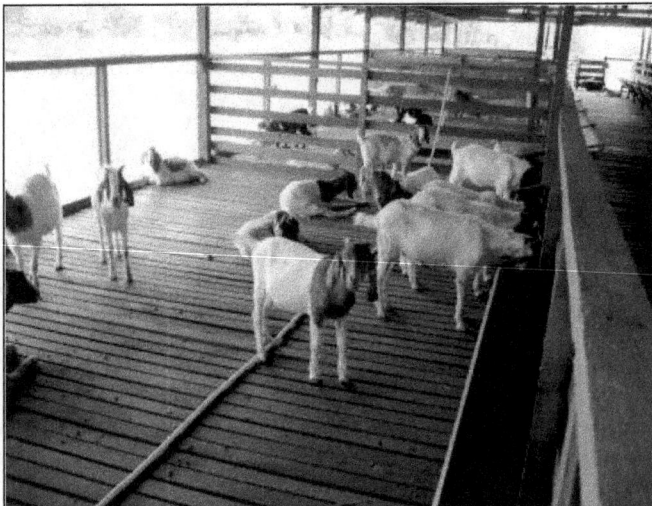

Elevated Flooring with Wooden Batons.

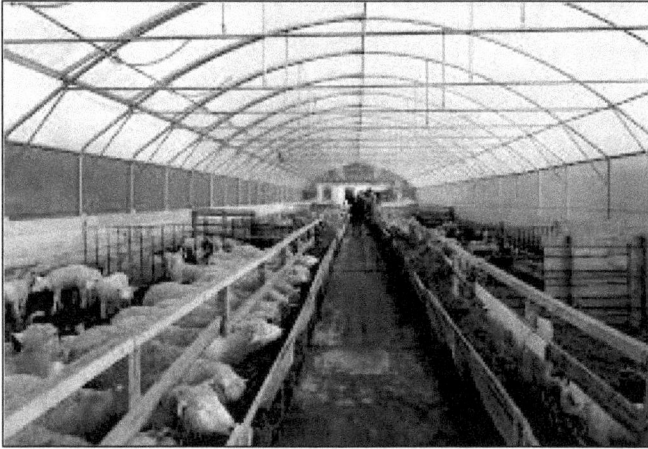

Length-wise Partitioned Shed.

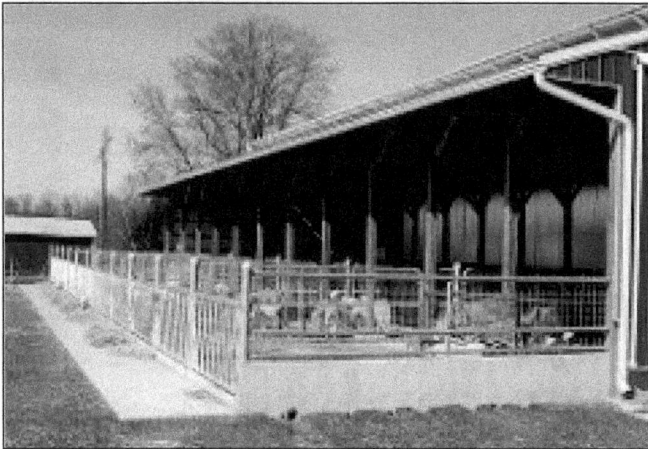

Housing with Run Space.

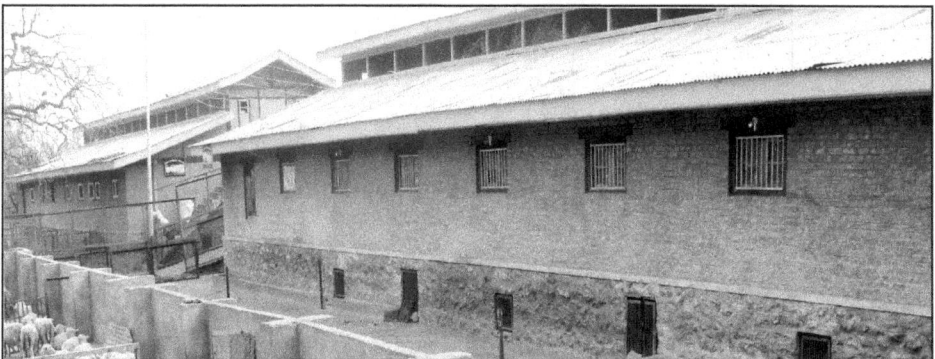

Shed with Elevated Floor, Run Space and Gable Roofing.

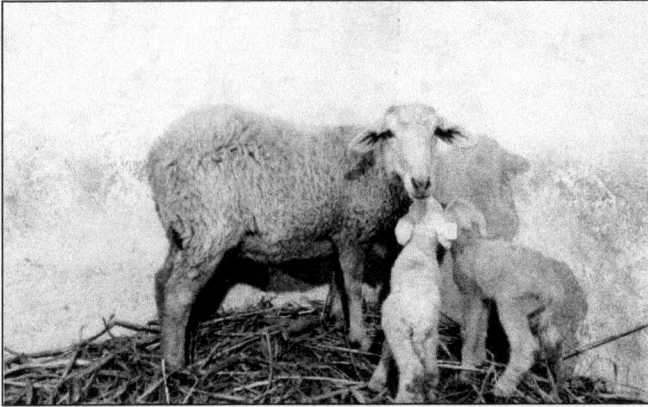

Lambing Pen.

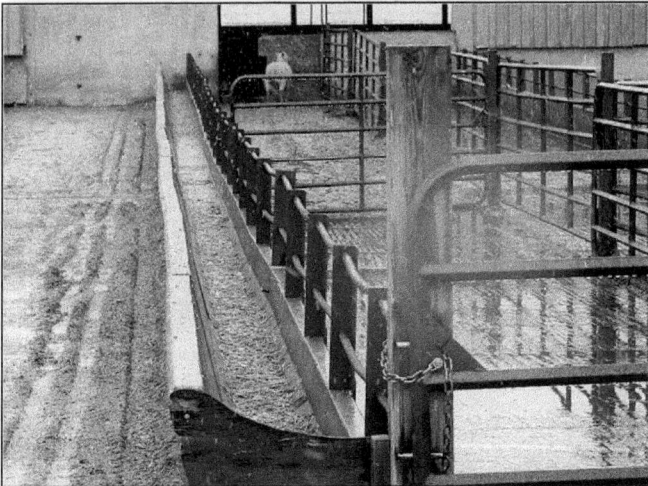

Manger for Feed/Concentrate.

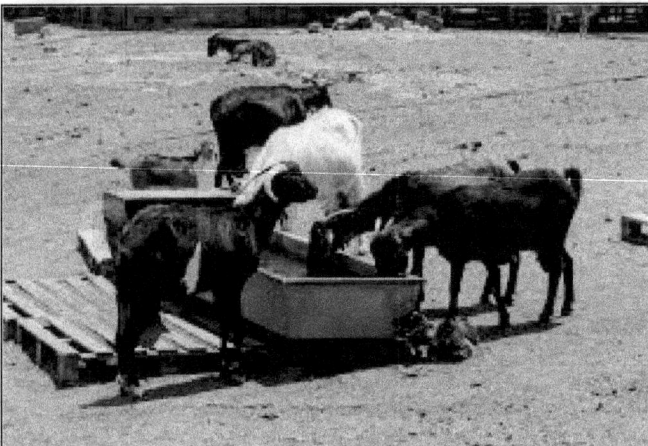

Water Trough.

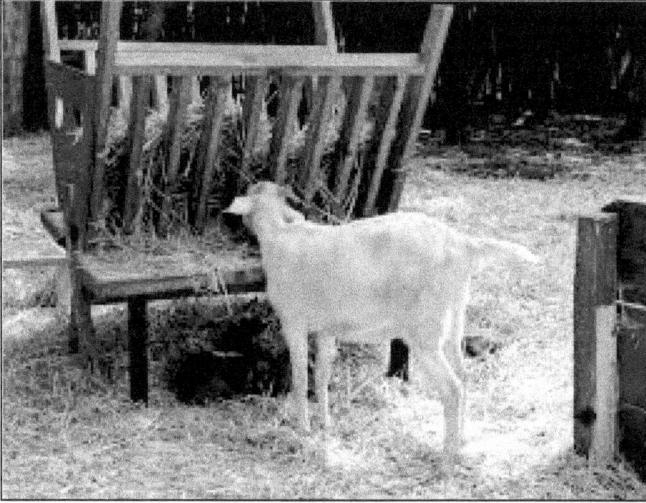

Fodder Tack.

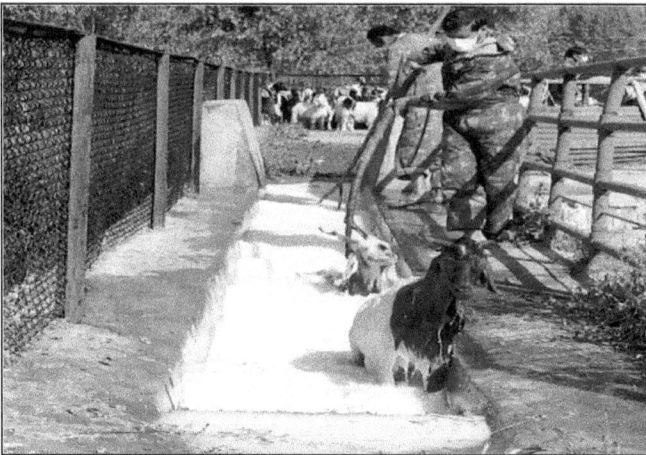

Dipping Tank.

Dispensary Room

☆ In an organized farm a dispensary room is must.

☆ It should be constructed at a convenient place in the yard with paca flooring and walls.

☆ It should have almiras and shelves to hold medicines and other laboratory items.

☆ It should have all required facilities available like refrigerator for vaccines and medicines, autoclave for sterility of surgical instruments and dressing material, dressing table or examination table for attending emergencies.

☆ It should be equipped with all emergency drugs, important medicines and surgicals, dressing materials, thermometers, stethoscope and infusion sets *etc.*

Shearing and Store Room

☆ The shearing and store room consist of two compartments with a dividing wall.

☆ One room may be exclusively meant for storing wool and shearing equipment and the other for keeping feed.

☆ The other room used for shearing may be 6m (l) x 2.5m (w) x 3m (h).

☆ There should be a door one meter wide and two meters high in front side of the room.

☆ This room should have clean smooth floors and walls lined with glazed tiles upto a height of one and half meter.

☆ The room should be made damp and dust proof.

☆ The store room should be also rodent proof.

Attendant's Room

☆ The shepherd's house meant for care-taker should be located at a convenient place in the yard to have watch and ward of livestock.

☆ The house may be 6m (l) X 4m (w) X 3 m (h). There should be a door of one meter wide and two meters high on the long side of the shed facing the passage of the yard.

☆ There may be many windows; one of these facing the passage of the yard.

☆ It should be suitably facilitated with water, light and heating for the animal attendants.

Hay Shed

☆ In a commercial set up you need to have hay shed besides feed store.

☆ The hay shed should be large enough to accommodate required quantity of fodder.

☆ It should be having concrete flooring with 1 meter height paca walls and net fenced up to 3 meter height to allow free air movement in the shed.

☆ Roofing may be of galvanized iron sheets particularly in temperate regions of the State.

Dipping Tank

☆ In a commercial farm a dipping tank is must to protect the animals from infections like ticks, lice and other cutaneous diseases.

☆ Dipping of animals is recommended twice a year in livestock farms to get rid of external parasites.

☆ A dipping tank may be made either of galvanized steel sheets or constructed of stone or brick in cement mortar, whichever is likely to prove economical, according to local conditions.

☆ If a galvanized steel tank is used, it shall be well bedded down and the soil rammed tight against it to prevent the sides of the bath from bulging when it is filled.

☆ The dipping tank may be at one side of the yard.

☆ It should have proper ramps on either side to allow animals going down in the tank and coming out of the tank smoothly.

☆ It should have a length of minimum 6 metres and 1 and ½ meter depth to ensure proper dipping of animals in it.

☆ It should be associated with animal assembly ranch and drying ranch.

Manure Pit/Vermicomposting Pit

☆ In a big commercial farm, manure management is of utmost importance to have clean farm atmosphere.

☆ The sheep or goat manure is dry pellet type and thus easily collected.

☆ It should be piled up in a deep pit, dug out in the soil at a distance from the farm house.

☆ For its vermicomposting, the pre-digestion of manure is must, which is achieved by keeping the manure along with grass/straw/hay in a pit and sprinkled with water and covered with polythene to allow its fermentation for minimum of three weeks. After that should be taken to vermicomposting pit of 10x4x2 feet and charged with the worms for compositing.

Chapter 3

Nutritional Requirement and Feeding Management in Sheep and Goat

Feeding management is one of the important concerns in livestock farming. Quality breeds do not express their full potential unless they are provided good nutrition and good environment.

In many animal production systems, approximately two-third of improvements in livestock productivity can be attributed to improved nutrition. In economic terms, feed cost accounts for about 70 per cent of the total cost of livestock production. The feasibility of livestock enterprises is, therefore, a function of the type of feed and feeding system.

Inadequate nutrition, particularly of energy, depresses the reproductive performance of extensively or intensively managed sheep or goats. Sexual maturity of sheep and goats is advanced by good feeding and the energy stimulates oestrous activity within the normal breeding season, ovulation rate, fertilization and survival of ova and the maintenance of the resultant embryos to term as viable lambs or kids. Body condition at mating, achieved over a longer period *i.e.* the period between one reproductive cycle and the next, has a greater influence on ovulation rate than flushing.

Intake and selection of feed and fodder does not depend only on the availability of resources but also on the feeding behavior of the animals. Knowledge of foraging behaviour and the dietary habits of sheep and goats (type and parts of plants they eat, their tolerance to saline or bitter feed and saline water, the distance of travelling to find food, the frequency of drinking and their walking ability) provide clues for development of managemental strategies aimed at increasing animal performance with best use of ecosystems.

There are six important nutrients found in feedstuffs and animals, namely water, carbohydrates, fats (lipids), protein, minerals, and vitamins which are necessary for life as well as production. Energy is derived from the breakdown of carbohydrates, fats, and protein. A major constituent of most feedstuffs is water. The other nutrients are said to compose the "dry matter" of a feedstuff and largely determine its feeding value. Plants contain mostly carbohydrates whereas proteins predominate in animals. Minerals and vitamins occur in relatively small quantities in both plants and animals. Feeds are classified according to the amount of specific nutrients they supply. There are two main classes of feedstuff; roughages and concentrates.

Roughages are bulky feeds containing relatively large amounts of poorly digestible material, that is, more than 18 per cent crude fiber. They can be dry and succulent based on their moisture content. *Dry roughages* contain only 10–15 per cent moisture and include Hay and Crop residues *Succulent roughage* usually contain more than 75 per cent moisture and include Pasture, Cultivated fodder crops, Tree leaves, Root crops or Silage.

Concentrate is a feed or feed mixture which has high amounts of protein, carbohydrates and fat, but less than 18 per cent crude fiber and is usually low in moisture. Concentrates are rich in either energy or protein and are thus expensive. They can also be categorized as

Energy-rich concentrates (Feeds with high levels of energy but low in protein content) *viz.* grains and seeds, mill by-products (*e.g.* brans, shorts) or root crops. *Protein-rich concentrates viz.* oil-seed cakes (by-products left after extraction of oil from oil seeds) and Brewer's grain (by-products of the brewery industry).

Feeding is done either to maintain the animal life or to have good animal production and reproduction. Maintenance ration is providing the energy to support essential physiological functions, maintenance of body temperature and body weight, repair of body tissues and staying alive. Whereas production ration is provided over and above the maintenance ration to get better animal produce in terms of body weight gain, fertility, lamb/kid crop, wool or milk yield. All these productive functions of the animal are energy consuming and unless additional supply of nutrients above the maintenance is not ensured, these functions will not be optimum rather will consume the body stores and tell upon necessary functions of life leading to malnutrition, debilitation and sometimes death.

In order to understand the fundamentals of small ruminant nutrition, we must first know the nutrients essential for growth, production, and reproduction. These essential nutrients are:

☆ Energy (fat and carbohydrates).

☆ Protein

☆ Vitamins

☆ Minerals

☆ Water.

The most common limiting factor in small ruminant nutrition is energy. An energy shortage will result in decreased production, reproductive failure, increased mortality, and increased susceptibility to diseases and parasites. The major sources of energy for small ruminants are usually pastures and browses, hay, and grains. Total digestible nutrients (TDN) is a broad term used to express the energy value of a feed.

In small ruminants, the amount of protein is more important than the quality of protein. When protein supplementation is the primary objective, the cost per pound of protein is the most important consideration. Protein deficiency is detrimental to the young animal, so an adequate amount of protein must be supplied if rapid growth and high production are to be obtained.

The essential minerals for sheep and goats are calcium, phosphorus, and salt. The primary source of these minerals is the diet, however, various mineral supplements are added to the ration as per the requirement. Vitamins are compounds which are necessary for normal growth, health, and reproduction. Small ruminants require many vitamins, just as other animals do. However, their dietary vitamin requirements are relatively simple because of the nature of the feeds they ordinarily consume and the synthesis of vitamins in the rumen.

Water is an essential nutrient both for animal welfare and profitable business. The quantity and quality of water (salinity, acidity, toxic substances) varies with the livestock species and classes of stock within the species. Its requirement also varies with the environmental conditions. The important functions of water in the animal body include

☆ Helping to digest food

☆ Regulating the body temperature

☆ Lubricating

☆ Transporting waste from the body.

Among the domestic ruminants, camels are true browsers, goats are intermediate selective feeders with preference for browse, sheep are nonselective intermediate feeders with preference for grasses and cattle, buffaloes and donkeys are grazers. Goats have been considered more efficient in the digestion of crude fibre and the utilization of poor roughages than sheep. Feeding of animals is also dependent on age and physiological state of the animal viz weaner, hogget, pregnant, lactating, breeding or dry. As per the needs of the animal feeding is planned and provided.

The energy requirements of sheep and goats are similar according to NRC (1981). For dry non-pregnant animals, the maintenance requirements are 0.42 MJ ME/kgW$^{0.75}$. During the first 15 weeks of pregnancy energy requirements increase by 15 per cent, providing also for a slight weight gain, and during the last stages of pregnancy requirement increases by 80–100 per cent compared with dry animals. For each kg of sheep milk (6 per cent fat) and goat milk (4 per cent fat) - 7.5MJ ME and 5.2MJ ME are required, respectively. The requirements for digestible crude protein range from 2.3 – 2.8g/kgW$^{0.75}$ for sheep and goats respectively for maintenance, which increases during the last stages of pregnancy by 80–100 per cent. For each kg

Some of the Important Facts about Sheep and Goat Related to Feeding Behavior

Characteristics	Goats	Sheep
Activity	Can stand on its hind legs to access browse; can walk longer distances	Walk shorter distances
Feeding pattern	Browser; more selective	Grazer; less selective
Variety in feeds	Preference greater	Preference limited
Salivary secretion rate	Greater	Moderate
Recycling of urea in saliva	Greater	Less
Dry matter intake		
For meat production	3 per cent of body weight	3 per cent of body weight
For milk production	4–6 per cent of body weight	3 per cent of body weight
Digestive efficiency	Higher with coarse roughage	Less efficient
Retention time	Longer	Shorter
Water intake per unit dry matter	LOWER	HIGHER
Water economy	More efficient	Less efficient
Water turnover rate	Lower	Higher
Water loss in Feces	Less	Higher
Urine	More concentrated	Less concentrated
Fat metabolism	Increase during periods of water shortages	Less evident

of goat milk or sheep milk 45–70 g or 60–90 g digestible crude protein are required, respectively. The calcium requirements for both sheep and goat are 0.623*DMI+0.228 g/day and phosphorus 1.6 (0.693*DMI) – 0.06 g/day. However, for each kg milk produced 1.2g calcium and 1.3g phosphorus is given additionally.

Feeding different Age Groups of Sheep and Goat

As already mentioned above the nutrient requirements of sheep and goat are similar, therefore, feeding in different age groups shall remain true for both sheep and goat. Some important guidelines for feeding different groups of animals are listed below.

Adult Breeding Males

☆ Adult males used for breeding need to be well-fed to maintain their body condition for mating.

☆ Breeding males need to be supplemented two weeks before start of breeding and during breeding season. They shouldn't, however, be allowed to become too fat.

☆ Feed them with Grass/crop residues, free choice (as much as they can consume),

☆ Provide legumes, up to 1 part for every 4–6 parts of grass/residue consumed or a handful (about 250 grams) of concentrate that should be higher (400–600 g) if the male is large and is serving a large number of females.

☆ Breeding males need to be supplied with plenty of water and allowed to exercise.

☆ Supply of good pasture is enough when not being used for mating.

Dry Breeding Females

☆ A dry female that has recently been weaned from her lambs/kids can be maintained on good quality pasture or good quality hay depending on her physical condition at weaning.

☆ Very thin animals that are adversely affected by the stress of lactation (especially those that gave birth to twins or triplets) need supplementation (handful of grains/concentrates) in addition to forage for adequate preparation for the next breeding and conception.

Breeding Females

Thin breeding females should be flushed before breeding.

Flushing is the practice of extra feeding the ewe/doe so that she starts to gain weight about two to three weeks before breeding. Flushing works best on females in poor body condition. This practice will bring ewes into heat earlier in the season thereby giving early lambs. It also has the effect of bringing the ewes into heat a more nearly the same time, resulting in a more uniform lamb crop. Besides, flushing also increases the lambing rate and incidence of multiple births in the flock. In J&K State flushing of ewes could be started from first week of August. Some of the suggested flushing rations are given below

☆ A good mixed pasture of legumes and grasses,

☆ A grass pasture plus 150 g of wheat bran per head per day,

☆ A grass pasture plus 250 g of grains and 450 g of oil cakes,

☆ Legume hay full fed plus 100 g of wheat bran and 150 to 200 g of grain and

☆ Green fodder at the rate of 10 per cent of body weight and 150-200 g of concentrate per head per day.

While taking good care of nutrition in breeding females, it is necessary to discourage the over-fattening that will result in reduced fertility. The over-fat ewes may be gradually brought down to the desirable lean condition, by reducing the ration and by exercising.

Young, Replacement Females

Young females selected for breeding, need extra feed for growth so that they will be large enough and in good shape for breeding.

☆ Provide young replacement females with grass/crop residue, free choice,

☆ Supplement legumes, up to 1 part for every 3 parts of grass/residue consumed,

☆ Supplement a handful (250–300 g) of a mixed concentrate.

Pregnant Females

Pregnant females need feed to support the growth of the fetus. They shouldn't be fed to become too fat. Females that are too fat will have trouble in lambing/kidding. Females in early pregnancy should receive:

☆ Grass/crop residue, free choice.

☆ One part legume for every 3 parts grass/residue.

☆ A handful of concentrate, 200 g/head/day mixed concentrate or 500 g of wheat bran.

Females in Late Pregnancy (2–3 weeks before the due date)

This is by far the most critical period during which correct feeding is important as the fetus grows fastest at this stage of development. In this period fetal growth increases 60 – 80 per cent until parturition and lack of enough energy in the feed can cause pregnancy toxemia in does. So during this period, animals should be allowed in very good quality pasture 4-5 hours per day. They should receive:

☆ Free access to good pasture and other roughage, crop after maths (crop stubbles), wild grasses and weeds or green fodder at the rate of 5-7 kg per head per day or good quality hay 3-4 per cent body weight.

☆ One part legume for every 3 parts grass/residue.

☆ Concentrate, 250–400 g/head/day mixed concentrate and 50-100 g molasses/day/head or 1 kg wheat bran depending on condition of the animal.

☆ 600 g of quality legume hay or 300 g of concentrate with 12 to 14 per cent DCP and 65 to 70 per cent TDN during last 45 days of pregnancy.

Lambed Females

Since the females have given birth to the lambs/kids they need good nutrition to nurse their young's.

☆ As lambing time approaches or immediately after lambing, the grain allowance should be materially reduced but good quality dry roughage should be fed free of choice.

☆ After parturition the ration of the female may be gradually increased so that she receives the full ration in divided doses six to seven times in a day.

☆ In general, bulky and laxative feedstuffs may be included in the ration during the first few days.

☆ A mixture of wheat bran and barely or oats or maize at 1: 1 proportion is excellent.

☆ Soon after lambing, the ewe must be given just enough of slightly warm water.

☆ As soon as first lamb is born, formulate the creep feeders with lamb 'starter' ration.

☆ An ideal starter ration can be 16 parts groundnut cake and 84 parts barely or maize grain and available green or dry fodder.

Lactating Females

The requirement of these classes of animals is similar to females in late pregnancy. Their rations should generally contain 14–16 per cent crude protein. They have high requirements for milk production. Ration for lactating ewes must be supplemented to maintain adequate milk production, which is necessary for rapid growth of lambs. They should receive:

☆ Grass/crop residue, free choice.

☆ One part legume for every 3 parts grass/residue.

☆ An average ewe's daily pasture requirements can be replaced 50 per cent by 450 g of good hay, 1.4 kg silage or 250 g of grain.

☆ Concentrate: 300-400 g/head/day mixed concentrate or 1 kg wheat bran. The level of concentrate should be higher for high milk producers. An allowance of concentrates at the rate of one third of the amount of milk produced is necessary.

The following rations may be recommended for lactating does

☆ 6-8 hours grazing + 10 kg cultivated green fodder/day

☆ 6-8 hours grazing + 400 g of concentrate mixture/day

☆ 6-8 hours grazing + 800 g of good quality legume hay/day

Young Lambs/Kids before Weaning

☆ Newborn lambs and kids should be supplied with colostrum within the first hour after birth. Colostrum helps protect them against diseases due to its high content of immunoglobulins, vitamins and other essential nutrients.

☆ Colostrum feeding is a main limiting factor in lamb/kid losses. For the first few weeks of life, lamb/kid needs its mother's milk and only that should be provided adequately.

☆ Colostrum is given at the rate of 100 ml per kg live weight. Colostrum can be preserved with 1-1.5 per cent (vol/wt) propionic acid or 0.1 per cent formaldehyde. Propionic acid is preferred for preservation as it keeps the pH value low.

☆ Hay, water and protein supplements should be placed near the lambs/kids after 3 weeks of age so that they start to eat and drink.

☆ Young ones can begin to consume other feeds at about six weeks of age.

☆ The creep feed may be started from one month of age and up to 2-3 months of age.

☆ They should be fed the best quality feeds available to help them grow and get them accustomed to eating feeds other than milk. The lamb/kid will increase its feed intake as the milk supply from the dam gradually decreases.

☆ The feed (creep ration) needs to be of high quality for their rapid growth because they can eat only small amounts. Generally, 50 – 100 gm/animal/day is given to the lambs/kids containing 22 per cent protein. Antibiotics like oxytetracycline or chlortetracycline may be mixed at the rate of 15 to 25 mg/kg of feed.

Ideal Creep feed can have

☆ Maize - 40 per cent

☆ Ground nut cake -30 per cent

☆ Wheat bran – 10 per cent

☆ De-oiled rice bran- 13 per cent

☆ Molasses – 5 per cent

☆ Mineral mixture- 2 per cent

☆ Salt – 1 per cent fortified with vitamins A, B2 and D3 and antibiotic feed supplements

Following Feeding Schedule can be Adopted for a Kid/Lamb from Birth to 90 Days

Age of Lambs	Ewe's Milk or Cow Milk (ml)	Creep Feed (gms)	Forage, Green/Day (gm)
1-3 days	Colostrum-300 ml, 3 feedings	–	–
4-14 days	350 ml, 3 feedings	–	–
15-30 days	350 ml, 3 feedings	A little	A little
31-60 days	400 ml, 2 feedings	100-150	Free choice
61-90 days	200 ml, 2 feedings	200-250	Free choice

Weaned Lambs/Kids

Weaning involves removing young ones from the milk diet to other forms of feed. This separation can be stressful. Lambs/kids are very vulnerable to disease and growth depression at the time of weaning unless they are weaned on to high quality feeds. Weaning is mostly done at three months of age depending upon management. Abrupt weaning is unnatural and should be avoided. Ideally, weaned lambs/kids should receive:

☆ High quality young forage - free choice.

☆ Supplementary legumes- free choice.

☆ Concentrates - free choice, starting with 70 g/day of mixed concentrate or 150 g wheat bran, and the amount can be increased as they grow.

Finishing

This is the process of feeding sheep and goats to slaughter weight with adequate finish (fat deposit). Intensive feeding of sheep and goats before slaughter is intended for the supply of animals of acceptable condition to the slaughter houses for ultimate export. These animals may also go into a finishing operation targeted at supplying the local market.

The types of feeds used and the methods of feeding will vary with economic and climatic conditions and the feeds available. The policy should be to utilize grazing lands, waste lands and aftermath of grain crops as far as possible and supplement whatever is deficient, with harvested good quality fodder, hay or concentrates.

☆ An average lamb may be fed 225 to 450g of concentrate mixture listed below depending on the grazing conditions.

☆ If there is plenty of grazing 225g is sufficient.

☆ In over-grazed grasslands they may be given 450g of the concentrate mixture plus half to two kilogram of good green fodder.

Rate of Feeding concentrate per Day

Body Weight (kg)	When Legume Fodder is Available (g)	When Legume Fodder is not Available (g)
Up to 12	25-50	200-300
12-15	50	300
15-25	100	400
25-35	150	600

Feeding Management

Sheep or goats are reared under different feeding management system and each system does have advantages as well as disadvantages. In the State of J&K, Himachal Pradesh migratory extensive system of rearing is old tradition of Gujjar and Bakerwals, taking flocks from subtropical Division to Temperate Division during summer and vice versa making best use of the seasonal pastures located in different areas. However, most of the farmers who have taken sheep and goat farming as an enterprise, observe semi-intensive system of rearing animals, wherein there is integration of animal and crop production. Animals are pasture or range grazed but also provided with crop residues, concentrate feeds or hay or roughages during the winter months. Intensive system of rearing sheep and goat is not in practice in the country which is a high input and high output system. Depending upon the size of flock, land availability and purpose of rearing, they are fed under following different management systems.

1. Extensive Grazing

☆ Grazing the sheep and goat in the entire pasture and leaving them there for the whole season is the extensive system of rearing.

☆ Gujjars and Bakerwals are keeping the flocks under this system of rearing. They migrate from one place to other and utilize the seasonal pastures without feeding any supplementary diets or providing any shelter to the animals.

☆ In this method feed cost is very much reduced.

☆ It is not conducive to making the best use of the whole grasses. So we can preferably practice the **rotational grazing method.**

Rotational Grazing Method

☆ Rotational grazing should be practiced under which the pasture land should be divided by temporary fences into several sections.

☆ The animals are then moved from one section to another section. By the time the entire pasture is grazed, the first section will have sufficient grass cover to provide second grazing.

☆ Parasitic infestations can be controlled to a great extent through practicing rotational grazing.

☆ Further, it helps to provide quality fodder (immature) for most part of the year.

☆ Under this system, it is advisable to graze the lambs first on a section and then bring in ewes to finish up the left out.

2. Semi-intensive

☆ Semi-intensive system of production is an intermediate compromise between extensive and intensive system, followed in some flocks having limited grazing.

☆ It involves extensive management but usually with controlled grazing of fenced pasture.

☆ It consists of provision of stall feeding, shelter at night under shed and 5 to 8 hour daily grazing and browsing on pasture and range.

☆ In this method the feed cost is increased.

This system has the advantage of:

☆ Meeting the nutrient requirement of animals both from grazing and stall feeding.

☆ Managing medium to large flock of 50 to 350 heads and above.

☆ Utilizing cultivated forage during lean period.

☆ Harvesting good crop of lambs/kids both for meat and milk.

☆ Making a profitable gain due to less labour input.

3. Intensive System-Zero Grazing-System

☆ It is a system in which sheep/goats are continuously kept under housing in confinement with limited access to land or otherwise so called zero grazing system of production in which they are stall fed.

☆ It implies a system where sheep and goats are not left to upkeep themselves with only minimum care.

☆ Intensive operation of medium sized herd of 50 to 250 heads or more oriented towards commercial milk/meat production goes well with this system particularly of dairy goats and mutton breeds of sheep.

☆ This system of management requires more labour and high cash input.

☆ However, this has the advantage of close supervision and control over the animals.

☆ In this system manure management is efficient and utilized as good fertilizer after either decomposing it or making wormicompost.

☆ Space requirement is minimized and more number of animals are reared in a small space.

4. Tethering System

☆ This is a subsistence family system and the animals live on kitchen remnants crop residues.

☆ Only a small size flocks of 2–10 animals are kept.

☆ Animals are tethered in a piece of pasture land and the length of chain is adjusted as per the requirement.

☆ Grazing is near inhabited areas and other supplementary feeds are also provided.

Strategies for Ensuring Appropriate Nutrition of Sheep and Goats include:

a. Matching Sheep and Goat Production Systems to available Feed Resources

One of the strategies of increasing feed availability is through increasing off take of animals through sale (destocking). It is recommended to sale out the matured and old animals and keep young, growing stock that utilize feed more efficiently. This will increase the available feed resources to the remaining animals.

b. More Efficient Use of Agricultural and Industrial By-products as Sources of Feed

There are various means of improving the efficiency of utilization of available feed resources.

Supplementation is one of the important strategies to enhance the efficient use of low quality feed stuffs. The main objective of supplementation is to catalyze the more efficient utilization of poor-quality roughages. Since the ruminant diets are generally based on fibrous feeds that have low digestibility and are deficient in protein, minerals and vitamins, provision of appropriate supplementary feedstuff during critical periods of the year is thus important to enhance productivity. This is especially true for livestock consuming poor-quality pasture and crop residue-based diets.

A supplement is a semi-concentrated source of one or more nutrients used to improve the nutritional value of a basal feed, *e.g.*, protein supplement, mineral supplement. Supplementation can enable animals to consume more forage, to digest the same quantity of forage more efficiently or to overcome a nutrient deficiency that critically limits performance. Grazing stock may sometimes be supplemented with hay or straw to provide bulk for prevention of nutritional disorders. This is when the pasture is very lush with high moisture or protein content or where there is a danger of bloat in legume-rich pastures.

Supply of small amount of Bypass nutrient sources is again a strategy to increase utilization of absorbed nutrients and animal performance. Inclusion of Bypass nutrients at a low rate in the diets is beneficial, these supplementary feeds are however, expensive and their use in ruminant nutrition competes with monogastric animal and/or human nutrition. This targeted use of supplements is referred to as "strategic supplementation" and is designed to have maximum effect and optimum economic benefits.

Supplement of bypass protein such as an oilseed meal, cereal bran, *etc.*, that should be given in amounts not to exceed 30 per cent of the total diet dry matter. Oilseed cakes and other protein sources that have been heat-treated have considerably higher proportion of bypass protein. A realistic alternative approach to supplying protein through oilseed cakes or other purchased feedstuff is the use of good quality leguminous forages as sources of supplementary protein. Legume-forages rich in tannins are superior as bypass protein sources since tannins link with proteins during mastication and reduce their degradation in the rumen. Other protein rich supplementation can be through Brewery by-products that could be available to farmers in the vicinity of breweries or Poultry waste in areas where intensive poultry production is practiced. Poultry waste can be either poultry litter or poultry excreta that are being recommended in sheep and goat supplementation.

Supply of necessary rumen-degradable nitrogen and other essential nutrients to enhance the capacity of rumen microbes to degrade poor-quality roughages in the rumen. One of the strategy could be supplementation of highly digestible forage, preferably legume, given at about 10–20 per cent of the diet. This helps to ensure a more efficient rumen environment for the digestion of fiber. The other strategy is to use urea as a nitrogen supplement in different ways like urea solution sprinkling of low quality fodder, or urea molasses liquid or urea molasses blocks to enrich the ruminal microflora for efficient digestion of fiber rich diets.

☆ As a general rule, if a deficiency is suspected, urea should be added at the rate of about 1–2 per cent of the organic matter in the diet.

☆ Do not include urea at more than 1 per cent of the total diet or 3 per cent of the concentrate portion.

☆ Do not use urea in creep diets because of reduced intake of creep diet or potential urea toxicity.

☆ Introduce urea into the diet gradually over a two- to three-week period.

☆ Feed urea-containing diets at regular intervals for efficient utilization.

☆ Urea can be supplemented to sheep and goats along with molasses in troughs placed in the grazing area. It is a cheap and simple method of feeding urea that requires low labour. A typical basic liquid mixture contains 1-part urea, 10 parts water and 10 parts molasses.

☆ Providing of lick blocks that contain urea, molasses, vitamins, minerals and perhaps other nutrients are convenient and inexpensive method of providing a range of nutrients, which may be deficient in the diet, that are required by both the rumen microbes and the animal. The ingredients are designed to provide a wide range of nutrients to cover all potential deficiencies.

☆ Feeding molasses/urea blocks (MUB) is a convenient way of ensuring a continuous supply of ammonia-nitrogen in the rumen, as is treating poor quality roughages with urea.

☆ Urea molasses blocks (UMB) have proven to be an excellent tool for the improvement of ruminant feeding.

☆ They are cheap, relatively safe and a practical means of supplying nutrients.

☆ They create an efficient rumen ecosystem which favors the growth of young animals and milk production.

☆ They also improve conception rates and the size of offspring.

The urea molasses block technology should be encouraged. The common ingredients used in making feed blocks are; molasses, urea, fibrous feeds such as wheat bran, salt and cement (a binding agent). Molasses is used to induce animals to eat the block drawn by its sweet taste. It also provides energy and some other nutrients such as minerals like sulphur. The block should not contain more than 40–50 per cent molasses or it will break too easily and take too long to dry. Urea, is used to make the blocks and its amount be limited to 10 per cent to avoid poisoning. Urea is essential in improving digestibility and providing protein. Cereal bran is the most common fibrous feed used. The bran provides protein and helps hold the block together. Finely chopped straw, bagasse, or finely ground leaves from leguminous shrubs *etc.* can substitute for cereal bran. Salt in the range of 5–10 per cent is added to the blocks to supply minerals and to control the rate of consumption. Calcium carbonate and dicalcium phosphate can be added to provide additional calcium and phosphorus. Cement is used to make the block hard. About 10–15 per cent is sufficient. Higher levels make the blocks too hard. Cement also provides calcium. Clay such as that used in brick-making can be mixed with cement to improve block hardness and reduce drying time. It can also reduce cost of making the block. Other ingredients can be added to provide additional nutrients. Oilseed cakes or brewery by-products can be added to supply protein. Trace mineralized salt can be used to provide additional minerals that may be lacking. Alternative ratios of combining ingredients to constitute various formulations of blocks are inked down (composition in per cent).

Ingredients	A	B	C	D	E	F	G	H	I	J	K
Wheat bran	25	25	27	35	40	40	23	25	23	25	25
Molasses	40	50	25	20	10	5	50	45	40	31	34
Urea	10	10	8	8	10	10	5	15	10	10	10
Salt	4	5	5	7	5	5	5	5	5	3	3
Quick lime	0	5	5	5	7	7	5	0	10		
Cement	10	5	10	5	5	10	10	10	10	15	15
Triple phosphate	–	–	–	–	–	–	2	0	2	–	–
Dicalcium phosphate	1	–	5	–	3	3	–	–	–	3	–
Oilseed cake	10	–	15	–	–	–	–	–	–	13	13
Clay	–	–	–	20	20	20	–	–	–	–	–
Total	100	100	100	100	100	100	100	100	100	100	100

Deficiency of minerals in the animals has reduced the productivity and supplementation of minerals improves production and productivity in animals. Using plants at a young stage supplies the highest amount of minerals to the animal as mineral content of plants declines with maturity. Mineral supplementation can be done through the use of multi-nutrient blocks that contain the deficient minerals. Ideally, specially formulated mineral supplements are provided in the form of a mineral lick.

Supplement during times of most critical deficiency of a nutrient, giving priority to supplementation of the most critically deficient nutrient. Make better use of supplements by giving priority to the physiologically most vulnerable groups of sheep and goats, *e.g.*, pregnant animals during the last third of gestation, lactating females, young growing lambs, *etc.*

c. Encouraging Increased Intake in Terms of Quality and Quantity

This will lead to improved body weight gain. Offering crop residues to goats and sheep at a 50 per cent refusal rate instead of the conventional 10–20 per cent results in increased feed intake. Such a feeding strategy of allowing 50 per cent refusal of the residue could be wasteful and is justified only if the rejected straw could also be utilized by less selective ruminants like cattle.

The widespread traditional use of browse in goats as an available source of quality feed during the dry season is vital to maintaining stability of livestock production in drier areas. Browse supplies goats with the bulk of their nutritive requirements and complements the diet of sheep with protein, vitamins and minerals. Foliage from trees and shrubs in pastoral areas provides more edible biomass than pasture. Moreover, browse remains green and high in protein content when pastures become dry.

The nutrient requirements increase with age, body weight and physiological state. The growing lambs or kids need more nutrients as compared to adults, similarly demands for nutrients increase exponentially during last few weeks of gestation or early lactation. It shall be easy to understand the increased demands of animal in different stages of life when its dry matter consumption increases. Increase in dry matter intake (per cent with respect to body weight) at different phases of life is squarely going to provide animal increased quantities of important nutrients like energy, proteins or minerals. Generally dry matter intake as percent of body weight in sheep and goat for maintenance does not differ much (1.75 per cent and 1.8 per cent respectively). For early weaners at a moderate growth dry matter requirement increases to 4.5 per cent of body weight, during last 4 weeks of gestation it raises to 2.7 per cent and during early 6 weeks of lactation dry matter requirement may reach to 3.6 - 4 per cent of body weight.

Nutrient Composition of Feeds Used for Sheep and Goats

Feedstuff Class	Dry Matter (per cent)	Crude Protein (Per cent DM)	ME (MJ/Kg DM)
Straws/stovers	88–92	3–4	5.5–7.5
Cereals	89–91	9–11	12-14
Grasses	20	10–22	9-12
Oilseed cakes	89–91	22–50	12–14
Green legumes	15–27	17–24	10–12

Daily Maintenance Requirement Estimates for Energy and Digestible Crude Protein (DCP)

Live Weight (kg)	ME (MJ/kg dry matter)		DCP (g/day)	
	Confined	Extensive	Maintenance	Pregnancy
10	2.32	3.25	15	30
20	3.91	5.47	26	50
30	5.30	7.42	35	67
40	6.58	9.21	43	83
50	7.78	10.89	51	99
60	8.92	12.49	59	113

NRC (1981).

Daily Nutrient Requirements of Sheep for Maintenance

Avg. Body Wt.(lb.)	Dry Matter (lb./head)	Per cent Body Wt. (lb.)	Total Protein (lb.)	TDN (lb.)	Ca (lb.)	P (lb.)	Vitamin	
							A(IU)	E(IU)
110	2.2	2.0	0.21	1.2	0.004	0.004	2350	15
132	2.4	1.8	0.23	1.3	0.005	0.005	2820	16
154	2.6	1.7	0.25	1.5	0.005	0.005	3290	18
176	2.9	1.6	0.27	1.6	0.006	0.006	3760	20

Expressed on 100-Per cent Dry Matter Basis

Avg. Body Wt. (lb.)	Dry Matter (lb./head)	Per cent Body Wt. (lb.)	Total Protein (per cent)	TDN (per cent)	Ca (per cent)	P (per cent)	Vitamin A(IU)	Vitamin E(IU)
110	2.2	2.0	9.5	54.5	0.18	0.18	1068	7
132	2.4	1.8	9.5	54.2	0.21	0.21	1175	7
154	2.6	1.7	9.6	57.7	0.19	0.19	1265	7
176	2.9	1.6	9.3	55.2	0.21	0.21	1296	7

Daily Nutrient Requirement of Goats for Maintenance

Avg. Body Wt.(lb.)	Dry Matter (lb./head)	Per cent Body Wt. (lb.)	Total Protein (lb.)	TDN (lb.)	Ca (lb.)	P (lb.)	Vitamin A(IU)	Vitamin E(IU)
				Maintenance				
22	0.63	2.80	0.05	0.35	0.002	0.002	400	84
45	1.08	2.40	0.08	0.59	0.002	0.002	700	144
67	1.46	2.20	0.11	0.80	0.004	0.003	900	195
90	1.81	2.03	0.14	0.99	0.004	0.003	1200	243
112	2.13	1.90	0.17	1.17	0.007	0.005	1400	285
134	2.44	1.82	0.19	1.34	0.007	0.005	1600	327
157	2.76	1.80	0.21	1.50	0.009	0.006	1800	369
179	3.05	1.70	0.23	1.66	0.009	0.006	2000	408

Expressed On 100-Per cent Dry Matter Basis

Avg. Body Wt. (lb.)	Dry Matter (lb./head)	Per cent Body Wt. (lb.)	Total Protein (per cent)	TDN (per cent)	Ca (per cent)	P (per cent)	Vitamin A (IU)	Vitamin E (IU)
22	0.63	2.80	7.93	55.55	0.351	0.245	660	133
45	1.08	2.40	7.40	54.62	0.204	0.143	660	133
67	1.46	2.20	7.53	54.9	0.302	0.211	660	133
90	1.81	2.03	7.73	54.69	0.244	0.171	660	133
112	2.13	1.90	7.98	54.93	0.310	0.217	660	133
134	2.44	1.82	7.77	54.92	0.270	0.189	660	133
157	2.76	1.80	7.61	54.35	0.319	0.223	660	133
179	3.05	1.70	7.54	54.43	0.289	0.187	660	133

Source: NRC-1981.

Water Requirement of Sheep and Goats

Sheep and goats should be provided unlimited access to fresh, clean, non-stagnant sources of water. Quality of water is very important which may be

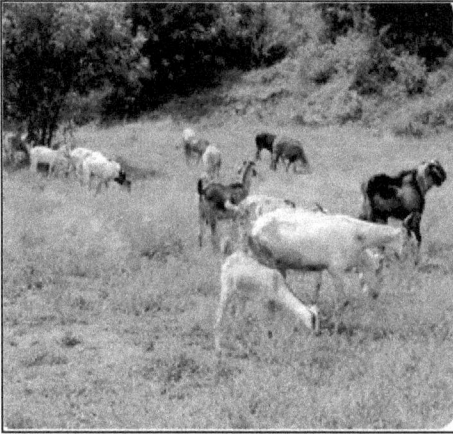

Extensive System of Grazing.

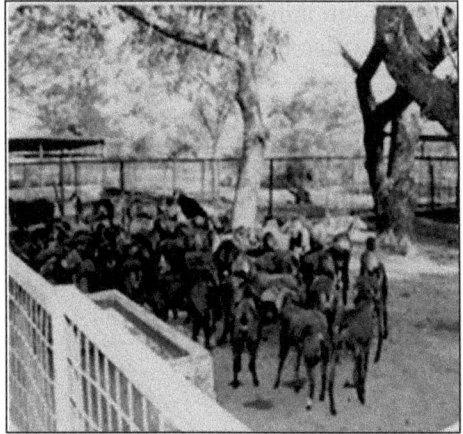

Semi-intensive System of Grazing.

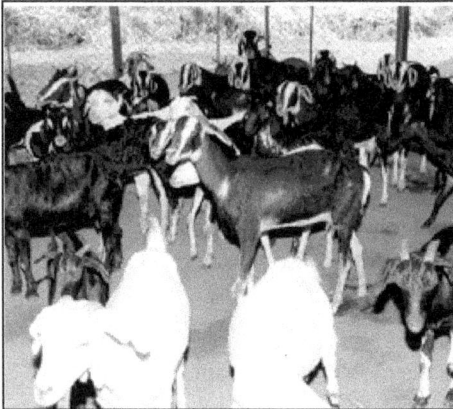

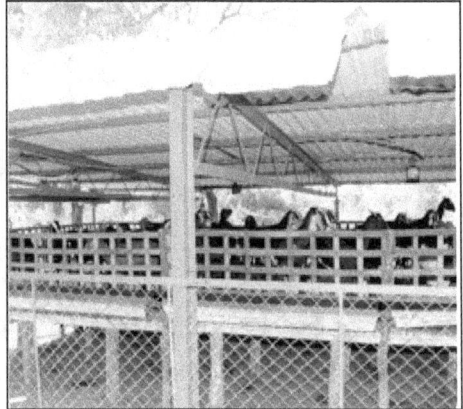

Intensive System of Grazing.

influenced by the salinity, pH or presence of toxic elements in the water. Salinity i.e concentration of dissolved salts in water should not be more than 10,000 ppm however, water with salinity of 5000 ppm is suitable for consumption. Similarly water with pH below 6.5 and above 8.5 is not suitable for livestock and may cause digestive disturbances. Concentration of elements like iron, magnesium, lead, arsenic, mercury or fluorides should not be much which will otherwise prove toxic to the animals. Water requirement may vary with the season of year, production stage (growth, lactation) and water content of fodders consumed. Cooler seasons of the year reduce water intake of the animals whereas hot summers increase water intake of the animal significantly. Water intake may increase as much as 50 per cent with an increase of ambient temperature from 15 to 20°C. Similarly grazing on lush pastures also reduce water intake compared to dry fodder/hay consumption because much of it is provided by the forage itself. Normal daily water intake is about 3 to 4 liter but it can vary up to about 10 liters depending upon size and activity (pregnancy, lactation) *etc.* Water intake may increase by about 75 per cent in the 3rd month and by 125 per cent in the last month of pregnancy. Below given table provides an estimate of water consumed daily by different categories of sheep.

Animal Type	Weight Range (kg)	Water Requirement Range (L/day)	Average Water Use (L/day)
Feeder lamb	27-50	3.6-5.2	4.4
Gestating meat ewe/ram	80	4.0-6.5	5.25
Gestating dairy ewe/ram	90	4.4-7.1	5.75
Lactating meat ewe plus unweaned offspring	80+	9.0-10.5	10
Lactating dairy ewe	90	9.4-11.4	10.4

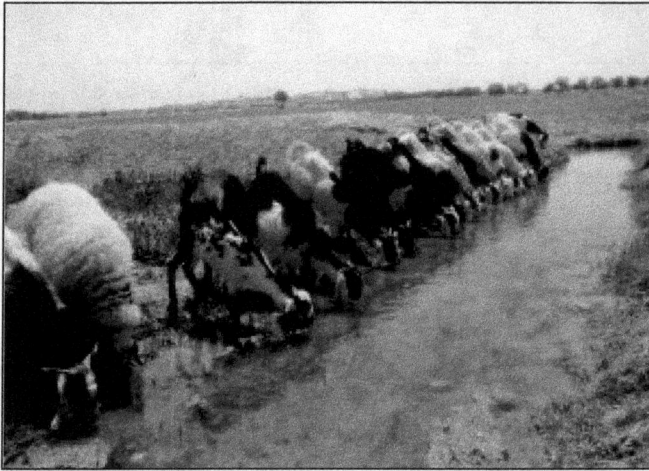

Flock Drinking Water from a Flowing Water Stream.

Chapter 4

Handling of Sheep and Goat

At times it becomes necessary to catch and handle the individual animal for its examination, treatment or other managerial operations. Proper handling of animals is indispensable to ensure the safety of the attendant as well as animal. It helps in making the animal docile, facilitates examination, weighing and even exercising of the animals. Handling of animals is also required to train the animals for show and competitions. Animals that are handled gently and are allowed to become accustomed to handling procedures will experience very little stress when handled. Animal stress is important in livestock production because stress reduces ability of an animal to gain weight and fight diseases. Stress also decreases growth, damages rumen function, and can interfere with reproduction. Reducing stress on livestock will also reduce stress on the handler.

Livestock (cattle, sheep, goat, swine, and horses) have broad, panoramic vision and very limited depth perception. These are perhaps the most important factors involved in livestock handling. It means that animals are able to see all the way around them, except for small blind-spots at the nose and in the rear, and that shadows may appear as "holes" rather than shadows. Panoramic vision also means they are easily frightened by shadows or moving distractions outside handling areas. Sheep, goat and cattle have a tendency to move from a dimly lit area to a more brightly lit area, provided the light does not hit them directly in the eyes. A spotlight directed on the ramp will often help keep the animals together moving.

Excited, aggressive handling causes animals to watch the activity rather than move in the right direction. Loud, abrupt noises, such as the sound of banging can cause distress in livestock.

An understanding of some behavioural traits of sheep and goat will make the catching, handling, weighing and moving of the animals much easier.

☆ Sheep is a herd animal and tend to remain always together and as such it is not easy to catch/move an individual sheep.

☆ Most breeds of sheep are naturally sociable; they stay close to one another. This trait is called "flocking instinct".

☆ A sheep which remains apart is usually ailing in some respect.

☆ Sheep tend to follow a lead sheep while moving.

☆ Usually a sheep will refuse to move if they see a human in front of them.

☆ They do not like to move towards direct sunlight, but will move towards light when in a darkened area.

☆ They will not approach an unfamiliar area without being forced to do so, but will usually enter an open gate or door.

☆ They do not like to walk in water or muddy areas, or on sharp gravel or cinders.

☆ They will rather crawl under a fence than jump over it.

☆ In range areas, only the psychological restraint that the shepherd has over his flock, or a good pair of sheep dogs, are used to control the animals.

Catching Sheep

If you have to catch sheep in a pen, use gates or hurdles to make the pen as small as possible. Do not get into the habit of chasing sheep around a pen. This is not only tiring, but is potentially dangerous for the sheep as well as the person trying to catch them. Compared to horses or cattle, sheep are not large animals, however, they are very fast on their feet and very strong for their size. Approach the sheep slowly and calmly from the rear and try to maneuver the sheep into a corner. The sheep will likely attempt to escape but will probably not move away from the wall. Individual sheep can be put in a small catch pen.

Catching of the sheep can be safely achieved by reaching three places;

a. Under the Chin

☆ Approach the sheep between its shoulders and flank (do not approach too close to the head, because it will allow sheep to duck away from you).

☆ Cup your hand under the chin and point the nose up to stop the forward motion. Be sure that you get your hand on the bony part of the jaw, not on the throat.

☆ Place your other hand on the tail/rump to prevent the sheep from backing away from your hand on its chin.

☆ If you are near a wall, you may wish to gently push the sheep against the wall to prevent sideways movement.

b. Hind Leg

☆ In case sheep are moving away from you, they should be caught byone hind leg.

☆ Position your hand just above the hock and move your other hand up to control the head as soon as possible.

☆ As adult sheep are still able to kick strongly while being held just by the leg, this method generally works best for young, lightweight animals.

☆ Never catch a sheep or goat by the front leg. This could result in injury of the animal.

c. The Flank

☆ Catch the animal by the front part of the hind leg as near as possible to the body.

☆ Place your free hand up to the head as soon as possible. If you control the head the rest of the animal will stay there as well.

Whichever method is used, remember that the wool is not a handle and should not be used as a means of controlling the sheep. This is particularly important when handling animals near slaughter weight, because wool pulling is a significant cause of muscle bruising and meat wastage. Similarly catching the animal by its horns is not advisable as it may injure handler and animal alike if horn is broken. The head should be held high enough to control the animal, or else it will be difficult to handle. Sheep and goats have much more power when their head is down.

Tipping/Sitting a Sheep

Sheep are easier to handle for administrating medicine, trimming of hooves, shearing or general examination, when they are put in a sitting position. The sitting position of the sheep can be attained by observing following simple technique.

☆ Stand the sheep in front of you.

☆ Hold the sheep's head in your left hand, placing your hand under the jaw.

☆ Put your left knee near or just behind the sheep's left shoulder

☆ Put your right leg touching the sheep's side near its left hip and your right hand on the sheep's back over the hips.

☆ Turn the sheep's nose away from you towards its shoulder you will feel the weight of the sheep against your legs.

☆ Take a step back with your right leg. The hind leg of the sheep will start to go down. Continue to bring the head of the sheep around until the sheep is sitting down.

☆ Some farmers will use a, "SHEEP CHAIR," to work on. This keeps the sheep still and comfortable.

Moving Sheep

While moving the sheep for pasture herding or in the barn, one need to take following steps for moving the sheep calmly and comfortably.

☆ When moving sheep and goats out of the pasture, it is easiest to teach them to come when called and to follow the handler.

☆ Calling them the same way each time and using grain in a bucket as an incentive with the leader/s is an effective and quick way of teaching them to follow.

☆ Sheep and goats feel much more secure following the same safe paths and routines.

☆ Consistency with feeding and or calling will work when moving sheep and goats. They will usually follow a bucketful of grain as well.

☆ Once they know what you want and where they are going, they will move right along and often pass the handler on their way to their destination. The handler should follow along quietly, with purpose and without stopping forward momentum.

☆ If you want a sheep to go backward stand in front of it. If you want it to turn to the left then stand to its right side and to move sheep to the right, stand to its left side.

☆ Sheep always will move the best when you walk behind them. Using a low voice and keeping the flock together.

☆ Move the flock slowly and quietly without exciting them and Keep the flock together when moving.

☆ If one or two sheep break away from the flock, try to hold the flock together; the strays will usually return.

☆ If the flock is to turned into a barn or pasture, send an assistant or a dog ahead of them to accomplish this.

☆ Sometimes sheep moving can be assisted by verbal ("up, sheep!"), a whistle, light hand clapping and physical prodding by hand.

☆ Do not move a sheep or goat too far away from the rest of the flock because sheep will become easily stressed and unmanageable.

Handling of Goats

Handling of goats in principle is not much different from that of sheep, however, observing following practices shall be advantageous.

☆ Handling of goats is relatively easy as they are neither strong enough nor aggressive enough to escape the grasp.

☆ Many truly tame goats can be handled with nothing more than one hand under the chin and the other hand behind the poll on the upper neck.

☆ Goats dislike being held by horns or ears.

☆ If a collar or identification chain is present, use it to handle the goat. Most goats will stop struggling to escape if you grasp the collar or chain and slip it up towards the base of the skull. Small goats can be held by holding one leg.

☆ If the goat continues to struggle in escape attempts, place an adjustable halter over its head.

☆ The over-aggressive buck can be controlled with a halter, collar and ring.

☆ Limiting the range of movement of goats, tethering system works well. Fencing can also be constructed of chain link or earth mound of 5-6 feet height. Barbed wire fencing should be avoided as it will catch and tear the goats' hide as they run into it, lean against it, or stick their heads through it.

☆ Tethering the goat involves the use of a collar, ring, several lengths of chain and a tether stake. The stake, which has a freely revolving ring at its top, is driven into the ground. A length of chain is attached to it and to the collar ring on the goat. As the day progresses and the grass is grazed away, another length of chain can be added to the existing one.

☆ Whatever the method of handling, the buck goat should be respected. He is dangerous and unpredictable, particularly during the breeding season. He is most likely to charge and butt you or rear up and thrash out at you with his front legs and feet.

☆ When given the opportunity to choose, always allow the goats to roam freely. Tethering is a very poor alternative to freedom of movement.

Grooming Sheep/goat

Regular grooming is not limited to just providing housing, feed or water, but some extra to ensure good health, better growth and production.

☆ Grooming is the maintenance and cleaning of the sheep/goat.

☆ Regular grooming can help to eradicate potential health issues of your sheep/goats in the beginning and prevent them from escalating.

☆ Grooming helps in keeping animal in tip top condition for show or competition.

☆ Grooming a sheep/goat also helps to observe your animals closely and it creates a bond between you and your animals.

☆ Grooming also helps to observe or determine whether your animals have any health problems or not.

☆ Grooming a sheep makes a world of difference and takes a little attention from the owner.

☆ Grooming is also time-sensitive, when you want to prepare an animal for a show, clipping or shearing must be done few weeks before the show so that the wool achieves the appropriate look.

There are several things to do while grooming a sheep. Since sheep have thick coats of fleece, the grooming process differs from other animals. Care is needed to keep the fleece of the sheep soft and bright. For grooming the sheep following steps shall help in keeping sheep in top shape.

☆ Place the sheep in a sheep blocking stand. This prevents the sheep from running away or making any sudden movements. Sheep should be contained in the blocking stand for the entire process. The process can be done in parts to let the sheep rest.

☆ Run a burr comb over the fleece of the sheep. The burr comb removes burrs and other objects stuck to the exterior of the fleece.

☆ Scrub the outside of the fleece with a fine-finger comb. The finger comb should touch the skin of the sheep to massage and relax the sheep. The finger comb also breaks up dirt and debris on the fleece.

☆ Spray water over the sheep using a spray bottle. Start with the body of the sheep and move towards the face.

☆ Wear a rubber glove over your hand and rub five drops of sheep shampoo into the fleece. Let the shampoo absorb for 20 minutes. Rinse the shampoo with water using a hose.

☆ Brush the fleece using a pin brush. This untangles the fleece while it is drying. Let the fleece dry for 3 hours.

☆ Brush the fleece with a bent wire comb. Rub the areas near the face, neck and head. That opens the fleece and soothes the animal.

☆ Trim the hooves of the sheep using a foot trimmer. Apply foot care medication over the hooves after trimming. Return the sheep back to the grazing area.

Fitting

Fitting is shaping your lamb or sheep's wool for the right body shape. Ideally, the animal should look muscular and not fat. It's important to find out the rules for your particular shows, as some require recent shearing or in-fleece, meaning no shearing. Your sheep should not have any cuts, nicks or ridges.

Washing

Before shearing the animal, a good washing is needed that removes a lot of dirt from the fleece that help in easy shearing and does not clog the clippers. Wash the animal thoroughly with livestock soap, making sure to rinse well with a hose. Dry off the animal with a towel or hair dryer. Once animal is dry, put her on the grooming stand for shearing.

Shearing

Cutting or shaving the wool off of a sheep is called shearing. Shearing doesn't usually hurt a sheep. It's just like getting a haircut. However, shearing requires skill so that the sheep is shorn efficiently and quickly without causing cuts or injury to the sheep or shearer. Most sheep are sheared with electric shears or shearing machines. Shear your lamb slowly and carefully. Once your lamb is sheared, put a blanket/ drape on her to keep her clean until she goes to the show.

A professional shearer can shear a sheep in less than 2 minutes and will remove the fleece in one piece. The world record for shearing sheep is 839 lambs in 9 hours by Rodney Sutton of New Zealand (2000) and 720 ewes in 9 hours by Darin Forde of New Zealand. Sheep are usually sheared once per year, before lambing or in the spring before the onset of warm weather. However, in J&K State, Sheep are mostly sheared twice a year, before onset of winter and summer, *i.e.* autumn and spring. Feeder lambs are sometimes sheared to make them more comfortable during the summer. Freshly shorn sheep need protection from the weather elements. It takes up six weeks for the fleece to regrow sufficiently to provide effective insulation. Shorn sheep tolerate frosts well, but young sheep especially will suffer in cold, wet windy weather (even in cold climate summers). In this event they are kept in sheds for several nights until the weather clears. Some sheep may also be shorn with stud combs which leave more wool on the animal, giving greater protection. Sheared sheep should be provided extra feed and fodder to withstand shearing stress and maintain their body temperatures, especially during the winter.

Since the sheep shearing is labor-intensive, other technologies are often being explored for more efficient wool removal. Australian scientists created a chemical method of shearing called "bio-clip." In bio-clip, the sheep are injected with a natural protein that causes the wool follicle to break and the fleece to drop off on its own. Scientists have also developed a shearing table so the shearer doesn't have to hold the sheep. A "robot" for shearing has been also developed.

Shearing can be done either by Blade shears or by Machine shears, however, it is important to have clean and safe shearing of the animal irrespective of device used.

Blade shears consist of two blades arranged similarly to scissors except that the hinge is at the end farthest from the point (not in the middle). The cutting edges pass each other as the shearer squeezes them together and shear the wool close to the animal's skin. Blade shears are still used today but in a more limited way. Blade shears leave some wool on a sheep and this is more suitable for cold climates. For those areas where no powered-machinery is available blade shears are the only option. Blades are more commonly used to shear stud rams.

Machine shears, known as hand-pieces, operate in a similar manner to human hair clippers in that a power-driven toothed blade, known as a cutter, is driven back and forth over the surface of a comb and the wool is cut from the animal. The original machine shears were powered by a fixed hand-crank linked to the hand-piece by a shaft with only two universal joints, which afforded a very limited range of motion. Later models have more joints to allow easier positioning of the hand-piece on the animal. Electric motors on each stand have generally replaced overhead gear for driving the hand-pieces. The jointed arm is replaced in many instances with a flexible shaft

Rooing

In some primitive sheep, there is a natural break in the growth of the wool in spring. By late spring this causes the fleece to begin to peel away from the body, and it may then be plucked by hand without cutting – this is known as *rooing*. Individual sheep may reach this stage at slightly different times.

Skirting

Skirting is removal of undesirable parts of the fleece from the rest of the fleece. Undesirables include bellies, top knots, and tags. High quality fleeces should be skirted. Following the skirting of the fleece, it is folded, rolled and examined for its quality in a process known as wool classing, which is performed by a registered and qualified wool classer.

Blocking

When showing a breeding sheep, block their wool rather than shear them. That means you card and trim them so that wool appears uniform. This is quite time-consuming, as you must card their entire body only after first washing and drying. After putting them on the grooming stand, push the card's teeth right into the wool, then lift up and forward. Once you're done, take the hand shears to form nice and even lines of wool. The exact way you hand shear your sheep depends on her breed and its show standards.

Hoof Trimming

Goats and sheep usually climb, jump and run all over the places throughout the year which mostly depend on the condition of their hooves. Trimming of hooves can be very difficult for you, especially if you are a beginner, so it will be better to get trimming done by an experienced person and learn how this process is done. Trim the over grown feet gradually and not all at once. After the feet of your animal are nicely balanced, trim their feet regularly after every 6 to 8 weeks. Look for any sticks or rocks lodged in the bottom of hooves and remove it. Look for any foul odors on their hooves as it may be case of foot rot. In lambs inter-digital wax glands get blocked and results into limping which can be corrected by applying pressure on the gland and release the contents. Trim the hoof's perimeters and try not to remove large pieces at once. If you see pink in the hoof, stop trimming as you are getting close to the foot's blood supply. Your animals can become lame if you cut too much hoop at once and over grown feet can also make your animals lame. For preparing an animal for a show, trim the feet at least a week or two prior to the show because too close trim, could make animal to limp which is not desirable.

Clipping of Goat's Hair

As in case of sheep shearing is done as routine practice in the farm, clipping of hair in case of goat is also observed to keep goats a part of a green lifestyle. Since the sheep do yield wool during shearing which has a good market, therefore, shearing of sheep is given due attention, whereas goat do have hairs which fetch no market. Although goats are pretty low in maintenance as far as grooming goes, an annual clipping is a good practice for all goats. Shorter hair helps goats stay cooler and allows sunlight to reach their skin, which drives away lice and other ecto-parasites.

While trimming goats, observation of following steps may benefit smooth clipping.

☆ Choose a day after the cold weather is expected to be over.

☆ If possible, wash the goat before clipping. Clipping a clean coat gives clipper blades the longest life possible. For bathing, use slightly warm water instead of natural water, because goats prefer to be washed with warm water. For bathing your goats just wet the goat, use an animal or goat shampoo and rinse.

☆ Use electric or battery-powered clippers. While clipping, check the clippers frequently to ensure that they aren't getting too hot.

☆ Spray frequently with a clipper cooling spray or oil as needed.

☆ Clean and oil the clippers between each goat, or more frequently, as needed.

☆ Secure the goat. Hold a baby goat. Put an adult goat onto the milk stand or secure her to a fence or gate with a collar and a short rope.Give some grains or hay for distraction.

☆ Start trimming from the top of the body against the grain of the hair. Clip the back and each side, and then the legs, neck, and chest.

☆ Press on and move the skin over the hip bones and other bony areas for a smooth cut. Move from the areas of longer hair to shorter. Use short strokes on the legs and to correct any areas that you missed.

☆ Use a 10 blade on the body. If you want the coat longer, use a comb attachment. Use long smooth motions to avoid choppy-looking hair.

☆ Clip the hair that hangs over the hooves.

☆ While clipping a doe's udder, use a 30 or 40 blade. Clip to about the middle of the belly and under the legs, lifting one leg at a time to get the sides of the udder. Hold each teat between the thumb and two fingers to avoid nicking as you trim around it.

☆ Brush the loose hair off and trim any uneven areas.

☆ Trim the side walls of the hoof and the heel down so that they are even and flat with the sole of the foot (sometimes referred to as the "frog"). You may trim the sole if necessary. Trim slowly and carefully until you start to see pink. Once you see pink, stop trimming, or you will cause the goat to bleed.

Brushing

Regular brushing is the most important part of grooming a goat. Brush your goats on a regular basis, except the feeding time. For getting mud and surface dirt off, use the hard brush and for getting out the less obvious soil, use the curry comb. A vigorous currying acts as a gentle massage and brings dirt to the surface. Use soft brush for finishing task and it also helps distributing oils throughout the coat of your goats. Try to feel your goat's body with your hands and look for bumps and lumps, if they have any, which could be wounds or parasitic skin infestation.

To keep your animal in top shape, you may need various grooming supplies, some of which are listed below.

☆ Sheep blocking stand
☆ Good clipper. hand shears
☆ Burr comb
☆ Fine-finger comb
☆ Rubber glove
☆ Spray bottle
☆ Livestock soap
☆ Lamb or sheep shampoo
☆ Water hose

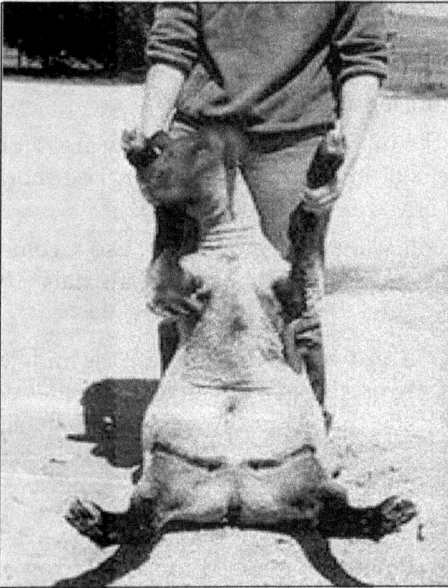

Tipping of Sheep.

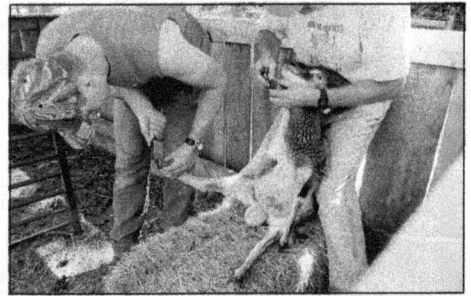

Trimming and Shearing in Sitting Position.

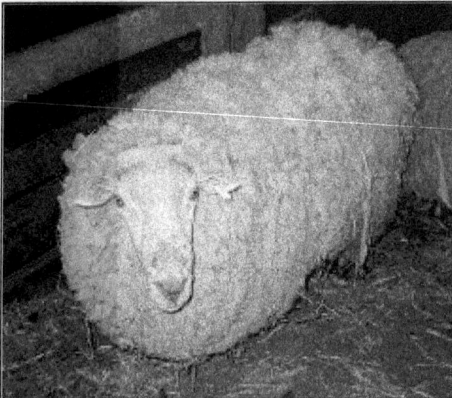

Overdue for Shearing.

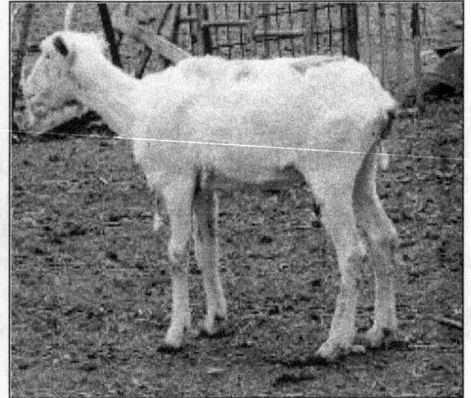

Freshly Shorn Sheep.

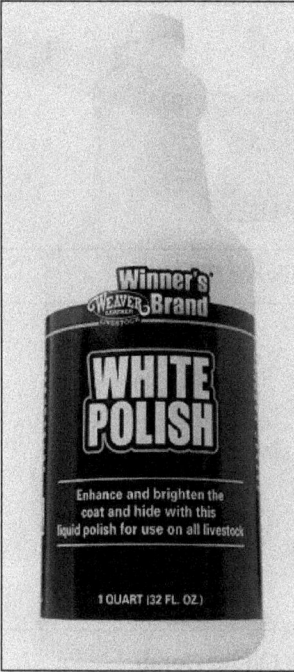

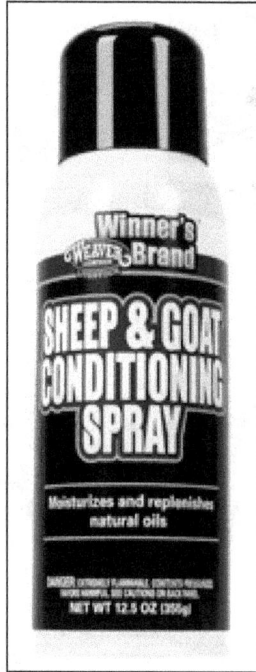

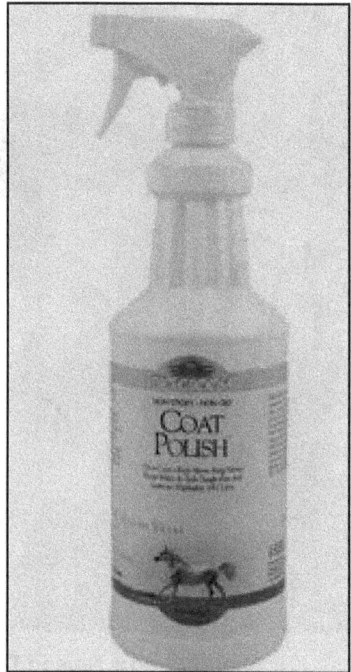

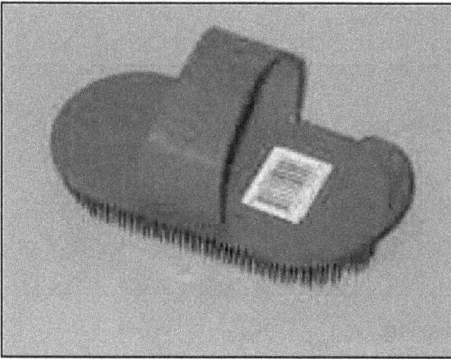

Massage Brush.   **Hoof Brush.**

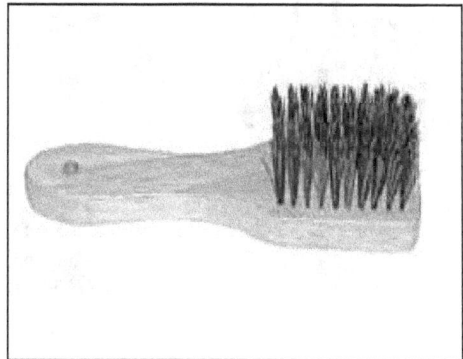

☆ Curry comb
☆ Wool cards
☆ Hoof trimmer
☆ Sponges and towels
☆ Halter and lead rope, teaching your lamb or sheep to lead.

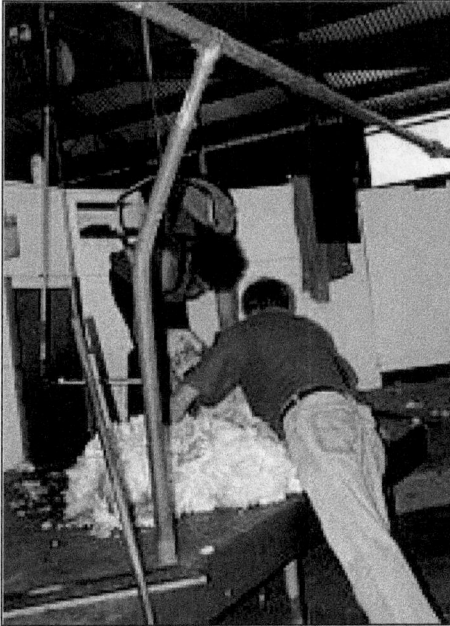

Slicker Brush.

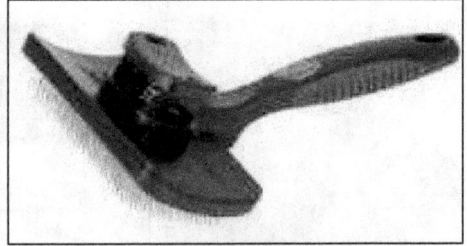

Shearing on a Raised Table.

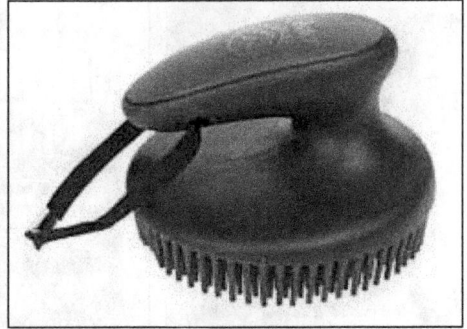

Fine Finger Comb.

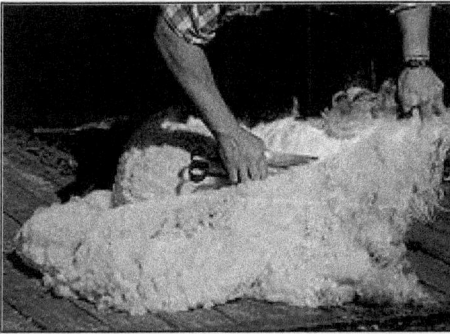

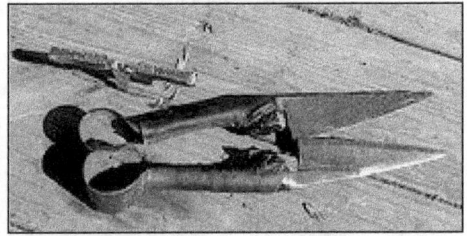

Blade Shearing.

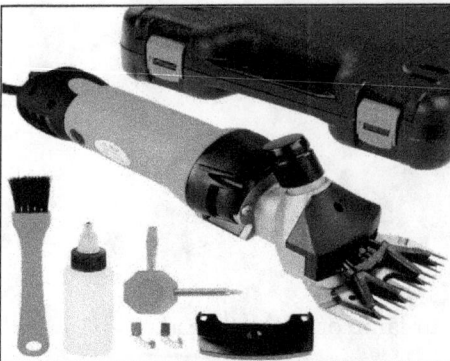

Electric Shearing Machine

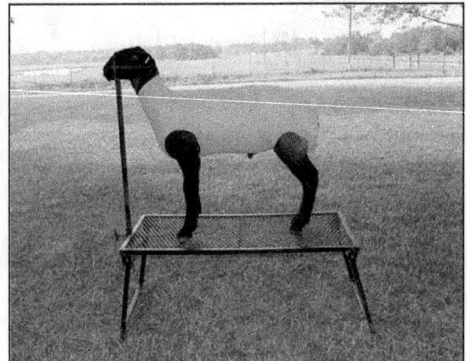

Holding Table.

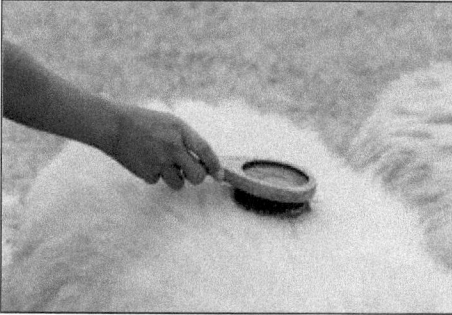

Grooming Brush.

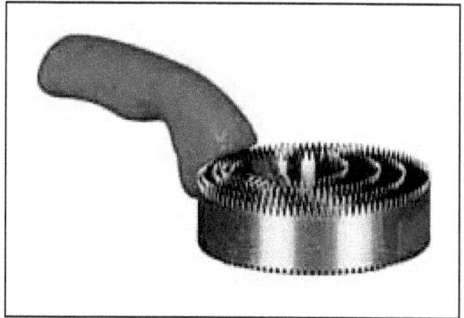

Spiral Curry Comb.

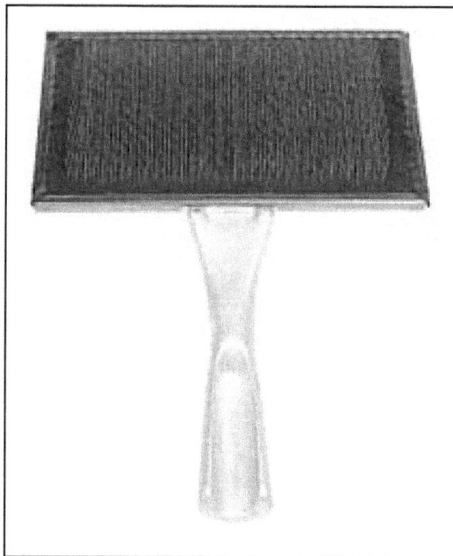

Card Comb.

Chapter 5

Management of Livestock in different Phases of Development and Growth

For profitable livestock farming, reproduction and production are two main thrust areas, wherein efficiency is must to be achieved. In livestock farming the crop i.e calf crop or lamb crop is backbone of its sustainability. In a successful farming the best young ones are retained in the flock as replacement stock to replace the old, unproductive or defective livestock, whereas surplus young ones are sold for meat or farming or raised to market age and then disposed. Therefore, for sustenance of a farm as well as increasing profit turnover, farmer has to raise lambs or kids to its optimum well beginning from its inception in the uterus of mother through birth, weaning to the maturity of the animal. Therefore, rearing and management of lambs and kids shall be discussed withregard to different phases of development and growth.

Care of Lambs before Birth

The care for lambs/kids begins when the fetus is in the uterus of the dam, especially in the last one third of gestation during which 70 per cent of fetal growth takes place.

Feeding and Management during Pregnancy

During pregnancy female is having extra requirement of nutrients to support wellbeing of foetus inside womb. Pregnancy is an energy consuming phase, therefore, management of animals during pregnancy warrants extra care and support. Supplying feeds of high quality during this period contributes immensely to the survival and growth of new born lambs/kids.

☆ As parturition nears, the dam should be fed supplemental concentrate in addition to good quality fresh forage or hay.

☆ Improper nutrition of the dam during this period results in small, weak lamb/kid at birth with little internal fat.

☆ Divide ewes into single and multiple bearing groups and also group separately the ewes with poor body condition and adjust nutrition programs accordingly.

☆ Care should be taken to neither under- nor over-feed animals during this period. Over-feeding at the stage may lead to difficult birth or 'dystocia'due to an over-sized fetus and might result in death of the newborn. It should be noted, however, that not all dystocia is attributed to over-feeding.

☆ Under feeding of the pregnant animal during last trimester will result in energy (hypoglycemia) deficiency that leads to a condition known as 'pregnancy toxemia' that finally leads to abortion and neonatal death.

☆ Dams that are not properly fed (malnutrition) will give birth to weak kids. The birth weight of such kids/lambs is usually below the average for the population. This problem is most frequently encountered in twin-bearing animals.

☆ It is recommended that ewes/does be provided with 50 g/day of concentrate per kg of metabolic body weight (body weight $^{0.75}$) starting from 90 days of gestation.

☆ Also use molasses in lukewarm drinking water @ 50-100 ml/ewe/day during last 1/3rd of pregnancy to avoid pregnancy toxemia.

☆ Add a coccidiostat to the ration 30 days prior to lambing if needed.

☆ Twins or triplets bearing mothers require supplying of extra protein and energy. Offering good quality forage and supplementation with 300 to 500 g/day of concentrate mix in the last 3 to 4 weeks of pregnancy is appropriate.

☆ Dam should be vaccinated for Tetanus toxoid and Enterotoxaemia 30-45 days before expected parturition so as to provide immunity to the lamb or kid when born.

Care of the Dam at Parturition

Knowing signs that are indicative of approaching lambing/kidding shall help farmer to provide appropriate care when needed.

The most noticeable changes are;

☆ Udder starts falling-out as the time of parturition approaches. In Boer goats, the udder can be very large.

☆ The attachment around the pelvis starts loosening and the vulva dilates.

☆ In advanced cases mucus secretion can be noted on the vulva.

Care of the dam at parturition include:

☆ In most cases, pregnant ewes/does do not require assistance during lambing or kidding, and is especially true if the presentation of the fetus is normal.

☆ When assistance has to be given, a veterinarian or experienced practitioner in the area should be called upon.

☆ The dam that is near to parturition should be shifted in lambing jugs where soft, clean bedding of grass or hay is provided.

☆ Lambing jugs provide privacy for the ewe and lambs to bond.

☆ Get ready lambing kits (Tincture iodine 5-7 per cent, gloves. Scissors, drapes, lubricants, cervical dilators like Epidosin, intrauterine lavages and boluses).

☆ When lambs are born, allow mother to lick.

☆ Dry the lambs with dry and clean drapes.

☆ Strip the teats of the ewe to remove the wax plug from the teat canal, wash the udder with antiseptics like PP wash and ensure lambs get their first sip of colostrum.

☆ Assist lambs in suckling the mother. If lambs or kids are weak take extra care in assisting them for suckling every two hours.

Care of the Lamb/Kid after Birth

☆ The first 24 hours of life of the newborn is most critical for survival. During this period, energy demands are high and physiological adjustment to the new environment is great.

☆ In most instances, newborn lambs and kids will stand and suckle within the first 20 minutes.

☆ Check for any abnormality in the udder of ewes/does.

☆ Ensure colostrum feeding of the newborns. Colostrum has many functions and properties, which probably makes it the most complete nourishment. It is laxative and aids in the excretion of the muconium, which is the first intestinal discharge of the new born. It has high nutritive value and, thus, provides an excellent energy source for the newborn. It imparts passive immunity as it contains antibodies (immunoglobulins) to protect the newborn until its own immune system begins functioning at about 3 weeks of age. It also provides warmth to the newborn.

☆ Lambs and kids weak at birth because of low birth weight, prolonged delivery, *etc.* may need assistance to suckle.

☆ If the newborn fails to suckle the dam, an alternative is to use bottle feeding. A small number of lambs/kids can be fed using individual bottles with rubber teats.

☆ Resort to artificial milk feeding or arrange foster mothers to disowned or orphan lambs. Goats can serve excellent foster mother but ewes which have lost their lamb early after birth may also be utilized.

☆ Lambs/kids deprived of colostrum will probably be sick most of their lives. Note that immunoglobulins can only be absorbed during the first 20 hours of lamb's/kid's life.

☆ Lamb or kid survival depends on optimum birth weight and intake of adequate amount of colostrum with high immunoglobulins.

☆ If lambing or kidding takes place in confinement, the umbilical cord should be shortened with a pair of scissors if it is long and then dipped in 7 per cent tincture of iodine.

☆ The untreated navel is an excellent route for infectious agents to enter the lamb/kid causing internal abscission or navel ill.

☆ Keep jugs warm with use of heaters or infra-red bulbs and have soft and clean bedding in the jugs.

☆ Check lambs and ewes in jugs several times each day to ensure ewes/does are claiming new-ones and lambs/kids are getting enough to eat.

☆ Do not handle lambs too frequently immediately after birth and let the dams lick and recognize them properly so as to develop a strong bond.

☆ Ewes with twins should be separated from those with singles. Extra care should be taken for twin lambs and ensure their udder feeding.

☆ Remove ewes and lambs from jugs after two to three days and place in small group of four to eight ewes with their lambs for further observation. Later combine these groups into a workable size unit.

☆ Screen the lambs for Entropion and Rectal-ani and get the conditions corrected by a veterinarian. Many a times in lambs there is impaction or occlusion or infection of interdigital oil/scent gland that results into limping and can be corrected by applying pressure on the gland pouch which releases the contents or if infected use local as well as systemic antibiotics with the consultation of a veterinarian.

☆ It is very important that the newborn stays with its dam for the first 4 days of life. This is essential to establish the dam-offspring bond. Lambs/kids are labeled by their dams during the first physical contact. It is, therefore, advisable to keep the dams with the offspring for at least this period.

☆ The milk-feeding period lasts from birth until the kid no longer consumes milk, accordingly, its duration is highly variable, lasting from 3 weeks in intensive systems or to 5 or 6 months in extensive systems.

☆ Start creep feeding in lambs above three weeks age.

☆ Give lambs vitamin E/selenium injections.

☆ Observe lambs for scours, pneumonia, or other problems. Start treatment for scours immediately after sighting problem.

☆ It is recommend that ewes and does with poor mothering ability be identified and culled. This trait is particularly important in free grazing systems where parturition occurs without assistance of attendants.

☆ Dock all lambs and castrate all ram lambs born during the previous week if not used for breeding purpose.

☆ Vaccinate lambs with ETV (multi-component) at an age of one month.

☆ Give anti-coccidial to lambs if needed at 3-4 weeks of age for 5 days and repeat it after 3 weeks.

Care of Lambs/Kids at Weaning

☆ Weaning is separation of off springs from mothers and disallowing suckling. The weaning period, defined by passage from feeding of milk to solids, is a critical phase characterized by a slowing or stoppage of growth or even weight loss. This is referred to as weaning shock.

☆ The level or degree of shock depends on weaning age and weight of the lambs/kids as well as the feeding program before weaning. Other factors contributing to weaning shock include sex (males are more susceptible to weaning shock than females) and health status. Healthy lambs/kids experience less shock than animals fighting a disease or infection, such as Coccidiosis.

☆ Age alone is not a sufficient criterion for weaning. In fact, in many instances weight is a better indicator than age. As a rule of thumb, weaning can take place when weaning weight is tripled of birth weight, provided that the birth weight is near or greater than the average for the particular breed.

☆ Weaning can occur as early as 4 weeks in organized farms provided the quality of solid creep ration is high.

☆ Every effort should be made to minimize factors that stress the lambs/kids, especially if those factors can be removed or minimized by management.

☆ The onset of sexual behavior in lambs/kids occurs very early, at about 3-4 months, so it is advisable to separate males and females at that age to avoid early mating and consequent growth retardation.

☆ The general opinion on weaning method is that if early weaning is desired, the process of weaning should be gradual. This can be achieved by restricting the frequency of suckling or decreasing the amount of milk offered.

☆ Vaccination of lambs at 2 -3 months of age against various common diseases like Sheep Pox, FMD, PPR, Enterotoxaemia, BQ or HS is recommended.

☆ Faecal examination of lambs should be done routinely to check any parasitism. Among many nematodes that affect sheep and goats, the most significant one is Haemonchus species. Most of these parasites affect the abomasum or small intestine of young, recently weaned animals and occasionally adult animals.

☆ Deworming should be followed atleast twice a year. Strategic deworming and tactical deworming should be followed after the screening of feacal samples of the lambs. *Strategic deworming:* This aims at reducing the frequency of treatment with anthelmintics and is used when most of the parasites are inside the animals and not on pasture. Treat lambs or kids at weaning and moving them to a safer place (parasite cleaned shelter). *Tactical deworming:* This is used to remove parasites from the hosts before they enter their reproductive phase and contaminate the pasture. An example of tactical deworming is treating animals 10 to 14 days after a rain.

Care of Animals near Matting

☆ Get the best sheep/goat flock ready for breeding.

☆ Do Breeding Soundness Examination (BSE) on rams and ewes like physical examination of udders and feet of ewes, scrotums and penises of rams, evaluation of semen characteristics if possible, previous history of any infection, abortion or breeding problem.

☆ Cull males and females that are not going to be used for breeding. Aged males and ewes should be culled.

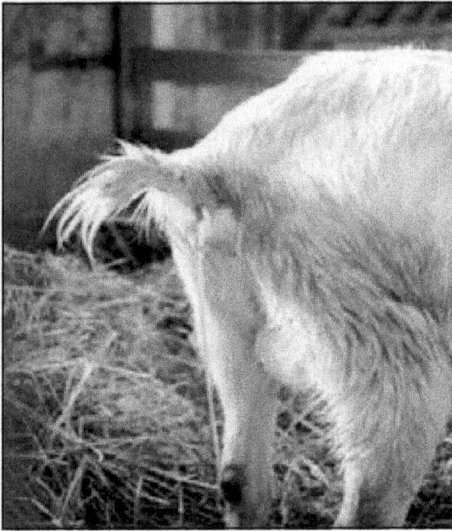

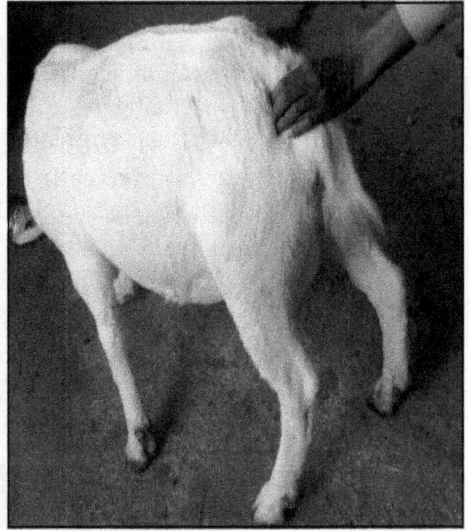

Signs of Approaching Parturition.

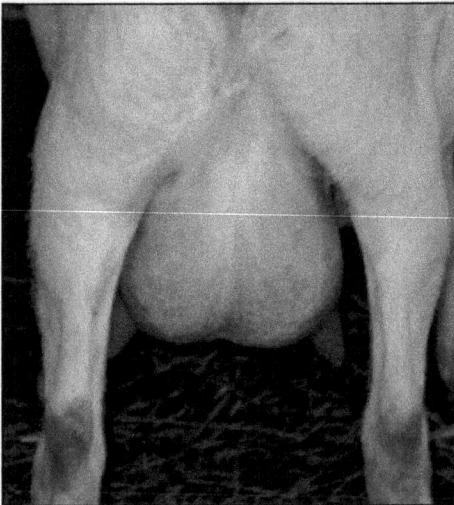

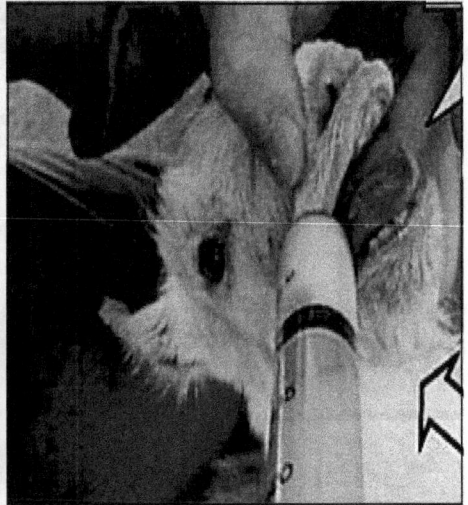

Bottle Feeding in a Lamb.

☆ Check Body Condition Score (BCS) and plan extra feeding with concentrate in poor condition males and females while sorting out in groups some three weeks before matting (flush feeding).

☆ Breeding males need to be supplemented two weeks before start of breeding and during breeding season. They shouldn't, however, be allowed to become too fat. They should be provided plenty of water and allowed to exercise.

☆ Feed them with Grass/crop residues, free choice (as much as they can consume),

☆ Provide legumes, up to 1 part for every 4–6 parts of grass/residue consumed or a handful (about 250 grams) of concentrate that should be higher (400–600 g) if the male is large and is serving a large number of females.

☆ Ensure mineral supplement (including selenium) daily.

☆ Do Faecal examination and deworm if needed. It is recommended to deworm the animals before breeding to increasing lambing percentage.

☆ Do use broad spectrum deworming agents after consultation of a veterinarian.

☆ Treat animals for external parasites either by dipping or by injecting avermectin/duramectin.

Chapter 6

Disease Control and Management in Sheep and Goat

"Health is Wealth" goes true with all life subjects be it humans, plants or animals. Animal production systems have remained backbone of livestock farmers and any health problem in livestock has a direct impact on production traits of the animal. In many situations where sheep and goats are associated closely with its owner as its family members and does feel pain if there is any health problem with these animals. Health of the livestock has much more importance in farming that farmer can only realize, therefore, proper health care of animals and management of diseases is an essential operation in livestock farming. There are many diseases affecting sheep and goat but their knowledge and proper management is necessary to keep livestock healthy.

Blue Tongue (BT)

☆ This is an acute infectious but not contagious disease of sheep and goat characterized by fever, inflammation, reddening and swelling of nose and oral mucosa, Profuse nasal and oral discharge, Inflammation and ulceration of lips, gums, buccal mucosa and tongue, and Cyanotic (bluish) appearance of tongue.

☆ It is caused by arthropod-borne Orbi virus in the family of *Reoviridae*.

☆ Biting insect of the genus of the Culicoides transmits the virus during the rainy season while blood sucking. Mosquitoes and other ectoparasites like sheep ked, *Melophagus ovinus* may transmit the disease mechanically.

☆ This disease mostly affects sheep and goat.Young sheep within the age group of one year are more prone to infection. Suckling lambs are relatively resistant due to their acquired passive immunity through colostrum.

☆ It is endemic in India. The disease occurs mainly during the rainy season particularly in the months of October, November and December.

☆ Transmission through semen and placental route is possible.

☆ The virus is resistant to decomposition, desiccation and antiseptic agents.

Management and Control

☆ Separate sick animals and keep away from solar exposure. Give adequate rest to the affected animal. Animals should not be allowed for grazing

☆ Wash the ulcers with physiological saline water or PP solution (1g of Potassium permanganate in 1 liter of water) 2 to 3 times a day and apply glycerin or animal fat on the ulcers.

☆ Consult the nearest qualified veterinary doctor for treatment and for ring vaccination in the event of outbreak of disease.

☆ Prevention of the disease lies in vector (culicoides) control with fly repellants. Use of ectoparasiticide injections is suggested in vector prone areas.

☆ Grazing of the animals should be avoided in areas where there is lot of vectors.

☆ Cloud of smoke with dried leaves/wood during 6 - 8 P.M. might help to keep off *Culicoides* from sheep sheds.

☆ Proper Vaccination of animals with regular intervals is must. First vaccination at 3 month of age and repeat yearly.

Peste-des-Petits Ruminants (PPR)

☆ It is an acute highly contagious viral disease of small ruminants caused by Moribilli virus of Paramyxoviridae family.

☆ It is characterized by high fever, loss of appetite, stomatitis, profuse serous nasal discharge accompanied by sneezing and coughing, gastroenteritis and pneumonitis. Oral necrotic lesions are noticed in lips, buccal mucosae, gums, dental palate and tongue, with malodour (halitosis).

☆ The disease is markedly evident in goat whereas sheep are less susceptible.

☆ Natural transmission occurs primarily through direct contact with infected sheep and goat, however, it may take place through contaminated food, water, beddings and other appliances. Secretions and excretions are rich source of virus and spread of the disease through feces may occur in epidemic proportion.

Management and Control

☆ Separate sick animals and keep away from solar exposure. Give adequate rest to the affected animal. Animals should not be allowed for grazing

☆ Wash the ulcers with physiological saline water or PP solution (1g of Potassium permanganate in 1 liter of water) 2 to 3 times a day and apply glycerin or animal fat on the ulcers.

☆ Consult the nearest qualified veterinary doctor for treatment and for ring vaccination in the event of outbreak of disease.

☆ Vaccinate the animals regularly. First vaccination at 3 months of age and repeat every year in endemic areas, however, it may be done every three years.

☆ Strict sanitation and hygienic measures are to be adopted in a flock. It is susceptible to most disinfectants, *e.g.* phenol, sodium hydroxide (2 per cent).

Sheep Pox

The disease has an economical importance as it causes losses from mortality, abortions, mastitis, loss of wool, skin condemnation and loss of exports. In ewes and does, severe losses may occur if the udder is invaded because of the secondary occurrence of acute mastitis.

☆ It is an acute to chronic viral disease of sheep and goats caused by a member of the genus *Capri pox virus, pox viridae* family.

☆ It is characterized by generalized pox lesions (crust, nodules) throughout the skin and mucous membranes. Soon after development of papules rhinitis, conjunctivitis may be observed. Mucopurulent discharges from eyes and nose. Animals die due to the development of labored breathing as a result of broncho-pneumonia.

☆ All breeds of sheep and goats irrespective of age and sex are affected. It is possible to infect goats with sheep pox virus and sheep with goat pox virus.

☆ Disease mostly occurs in April- June.

☆ Dried scabs, saliva, faeces, nasal secretions from sick animals for 1-2 months may be the source for spread of virus that remains viable for as long as six months. Usual mode of transmission is from direct contact with the infected animal. The biting insects (mechanical vectors) may inoculate the virus intradermal or subcutaneously.

☆ Virus is susceptible to highly alkaline or acid pH, to 56 °c for 2 hrs and 65 °c for 30 minutes.

Management and Control

☆ Isolate infected herds and sick animals for at least 45 days after recovery.

☆ Use disinfectants like ether (20 per cent), chloroform and formalin (1 per cent), phenol (2 per cent) to prevent the transmission of disease.

☆ Strict sanitary measures and proper disposal of cadavers and products must be adopted.

☆ Regular vaccination of animals with sheep pox vaccine – live or attenuated. First vaccination at 3 months of age and repeat yearly.

Tetanus

☆ It is a non-contagious, infectious disease of mammals caused by bacterial toxin of a strict anaerobic, spore forming bacteria *Clostridium tetani* which remain in the intestine of the herbivorous animals as normal habitat.

☆ It is characterized by spasmodic contraction of skeletal muscles. Stiff gait, restricted movement, difficulty in walk, lack of coordination, muscular stiffness and apathy to feed are the initial sign of the disease. It progresses through rigidity of the facial muscles with an anxious expression, 'lock-jaw', dribbling of saliva from the mouth, stiffness of muscles of the limbs with extended back and neck arched, erection and immobility of the ears characteristic "wodden horse stance" and sudden death within 2-4 days.

☆ Sheep and goat are more susceptible than cattle.

☆ The spores of the bacteria are very much resistant and can persist in the soil even for years. Organisms may continue to live in the faeces for a long period of time and thus remain as a potential source of infection to man and animals. The organisms gain entrance through deep punctured wound contaminated with bacterial spores. Organisms may gain access during parturition and manual handling of the genitalia with contaminants, retention of placenta and prolapse, castration by open method, shearing, docking, wounds by penetrating objects.

Management and Control

☆ Proper vaccination at day one should be used. Practice two doses of vaccine at least four weeks apart. An annual booster dose is recommended.

☆ Vaccination of pregnant ewes a few weeks before lambing is recommended that provides passive immunity to the lambs.

☆ Tetanus toxoid vaccines at the times of exposure of body tissues to environment through wounds or cuts is suggested.

☆ Cleanliness and proper hygienic measures are must to be adopted at the time of parturition, following parturition or at any surgical intervention. Similarly proper hygiene at manipulation of retention of placenta or prolapses or naval cut or castrations should be observed strictly.

☆ Sterile surgical instruments must be used at the time of surgical interventions.

☆ The animal should be kept away from metallic and sharp objects.

Caseous Lymphadenitis

☆ It is an important disease of sheep and goat occurring mostly among sheep producing countries in the world. It is caused by *Corynebacterium pseudo tuberculosis*.

☆ It is characterized by palpable enlargement of one or more of the superficial lymph nodes and most commonly affected are the sub maxillary, prescapular, pre-femoral, supra-mammary and popliteal nodes. The abscesses commonly rupture and creamy to caseated pus is discharged, with no odor.

☆ Source of infection is the discharges from ruptured abscessed superficial lymph nodes and the nasal and oral secretions from animals with pulmonary abscesses draining into the bronchial tree.

☆ Infection of an animal is facilitated by the presence of skin wounds but the organism can invade through intact skin. Transmission is by direct contact with infective discharges or mediated by contaminated shearing equipment, shearing sheds, holding pens, dipping tanks or yards.

Management and Control

☆ Management of the disease lies in high hygiene and proper sanitation in the sheds.

☆ The affected animals should be segregated and managed separately.

☆ Proper cleaning and disinfecting of ruptured abscesses is must to limit the disease.

☆ Administration of antibiotics with consultation of a veterinarian should be observed. The organism is susceptible to antibiotics other than the amino glycoside group.

Contagious Ecthyma (Contagious Pustular Dermatitis, ORF)

☆ It is a contagious viral disease caused by Orf virus of Genus Parapox virus, primarily affecting young lambs and kids. Morbidity may reach 100 per cent and case fatality rate 5-15 per cent.

☆ It rapidly spreads in flock by contact or via inanimate objects such as feed troughs, ear tag equipment, scabs *etc.*

☆ It is characterized by papules, pustules, scabs covering ulceration, granulation, proliferation and inflammation initially at oral mucocutaneous junction, oral commissures and spread to muzzle, oral cavity. Lambs cannot suck or graze. There is profuse salivation, lacrimation accompanied by nasal discharge.

☆ Malignant form occurs with invasion of alimentary tract. Severe systemic reaction can occur and lesions on coronets, ears, anus, and vulva can develop.

☆ Lesions can be multifocal in goats

Management and Control

☆ Affected animal should be segregated and strict hygienic and sanitary measures are to be adopted.

☆ The pustules should be washed with normal saline or potassium permanganate solution 3-4 times a day.

☆ Boro-glycerine painting of affected areas is recommended.

☆ Assistance in suckling may be needed.

☆ Lambs should be vaccinated when one month old followed by a second vaccination 2-3 months later is suggested.

☆ Non immunized lambs should be vaccinated before entering infected feedlots.

Infectious Foot Rot Disease

☆ It is an important disease of sheep of all ages caused by *Dichelobacter* (*Bacteroides*) *nodosus*. *F. necrophorum* aids *D. nodosus* in the invasion of the foot and contributes to inflammatory reaction.

☆ It is common in all countries where there are large numbers of sheep, except that it does not occur in arid and semi-arid areas unless the sheep have access to wet areas such as sub irrigated swales.

☆ Sheep are the species principally affected but goats are also susceptible. Older lambs have more severe lesions.

☆ It is characterized by sudden onset of lameness of several sheep associated with severe pain and sheep will limp or carry the affected leg. Usually more than one foot is affected and affected sheep may graze on their knees.

☆ On close examination the earliest sign of virulent foot rot is swelling and moistness of the skin of the interdigital cleft and a parboiled and pitted appearance at the skin-horn junction in the cleft that progresses to separation of the skin-horn junction at the axial surface just anterior to the bulb of the heel and proceeds down the axial surface and forwards and backwards.

☆ There is a distinctive, foul-smelling exudate, which is always small in amount.

☆ The source of infection of D. nodosus is discharge from the active or chronic infection in the feet of affected animals particularly the sheep. The organism does not survive in the environment for more than a few days, but it can survive virtually indefinitely in lesions on chronically infected feet.

☆ Infection into a flock can occur from the environment when foot rot-free sheep use yards, roads, or trucks that have been used by foot rot-infected sheep in the immediate past.

☆ Climatic conditions are major determinants for the transmission of foot rot, like moistness of the pasture and environmental temperature. Conditions of wetness and warmth favor persistence of the bacteria in pasture and increase susceptibility of the feet to injury and dermatitis, thus facilitating spread of the disease and outbreaks may occur in spring or autumn.

Management and Control

☆ Proper foot hygiene of the animal is must particularly when they are grazing lush, irrigated pastures. Any practice that concentrates sheep in small areas should be discouraged as it favors spread of the disease.

☆ The treatment of foot rot has been the application of topical bactericidal agents to the foot. Local applications include chloramphenicol (10 per cent tincture in methylated spirits or propylene glycol), oxytetracycline (5 per cent tincture in methylated spirits), cetyltrimethyl ammonium bromide or cetrimide, zinc sulfate (10 per cent solution), copper sulfate (10 per cent solution) and dichlorophen as a 10 per cent solution in either diacetone alcohol or ethyl alcohol.

☆ Foot bathing is a more practical approach to topical treatment particularly when dealing with large numbers of sheep. Copper sulfate solution (5 per cent) Formalin solution (5 per cent) or Zinc sulfate solution (10-20 per cent) is an effective treatment of foot rot.

☆ Foot rot can be treated with antibiotics without the necessity of trimming of the feet and is more effective when the sheep are kept on dry floors for 24 h after treatment.

☆ Vaccination against foot rot can significantly increase short-term resistance to infection however not yet available in the market.

Anthrax

☆ An important acute fatal disease of animals caused by a spore forming bacteria *Bacillus anthracis.*

☆ It is characterized by high fever, oedema under the neck, brisket region, thorax, abdomen and sudden death within 48 hrs of illness of animal. Following death there is oozing of blood from the natural orifices.

☆ When the case is suspected for anthrax, do not open the dead body. Dead body should be destroyed by deep burial with quick lime.

☆ This disease should be brought under the notice of the regulatory officials in case of an outbreak.

Management and Control

☆ Periodical and regular vaccination of the flock should be done.

☆ Strict quarantine measures in anthrax prone areas must be observed.

☆ Care should be taken to destroy the dead body by deep burial with quick lime.

☆ Persons handling the anthrax infected animals should adopt adequate sanitary measures.

☆ The adjacent areas of the dead and infected animals should be thoroughly disinfected by 10 per cent caustic soda or 10 per cent formalin.

☆ The fodder from infected pasture should be destroyed and not to be given to the other animals.

Pneumonic Pasteurellosis in Sheep and Goat

☆ It is a bacterial disease caused by *Pasteurella haemolytica*, predisposed by stress like, shearing, long journeys, malnutrition *etc*. The organism is natural inhabitant of respiratory tract, however, may be present on grass and in water in grazing areas and in the bedding of sheep pens.

☆ It is characterized by sudden death in lambs whereas adult sheep show signs of respiratory distress, dyspnea, slight frothing at the mouth, cough, and nasal discharge with high fever, depression and anorexia.

☆ Lambs are most susceptible during the first few months of life and ewes are most susceptible at lambing. Outbreaks often start with sudden death in lambs from septicemic pasteurellosis and progress to pneumonic pasteurellosis in the ewes and also in the lambs as they get older.

Management and Control

☆ Segregate the sick animal. Observe high hygiene and disinfection.

☆ With the consultation of veterinarian use antibiotics, commonly penicillin however, oxytetracycline, may be the drug of choice.

Clostridial Diseases

These are the diseases caused by toxin producing, anaerobic Clostridial bacteria. Clostridia are commonly present in soils rich in humus and multiply in soil in warm weather following heavy rain. Of major importance in farm animals are diseases like Black leg, Braxy, Enterotoxemia, Bacillary haemoglobinurea, Pulpy kidney *etc*.

Black Leg

☆ It is caused by *Cl. chauvoei* which is enzootic in flood soils.

☆ It causes Colostridial myositis of skeletal muscles.

☆ It is characterized by stiff gait, lameness, gaseous crepitation when the thigh muscles are infected, high fever, anorexia, depression and death.

☆ The disease is transmitted through wound-shearing, docking navel at birth, at lambing injury to vulva, vagina or fighting. Occurs mostly in warm months.

Braxy

☆ It is caused by *Cl. septicum*.

☆ It is characterized by abomasitis, toxemia, fever, depression, anorexia, abdomen distended with gas and high mortality rate.

☆ Lambs are found dead in morning.

Bacillary Hemoglobinuria

☆ It is caused by *Cl. haemolyticum*.

☆ It produces toxins in liver.

☆ It is characterized by toxemia, vascular damage, intravascular haemolysis, fever, abdominal pain, arched back posture.

Enterotoxaemia

☆ It is caused by *Cl. perfringens*.

☆ It produces number of toxins in intestinal tract of domestic animals that result in enteric and histotoxic disease.

☆ *Cl. perfringens* isolates are classified into five types, types A-E, depending on their ability to produce the four major lethal toxins: the alpha, beta, epsilon, and iota toxins.

☆ *Cl. perfringens type A* produces primarily alpha toxin, which possesses phospholipase C and sphingomyelinase activity and consequently hemolytic action and cause **Hemorrhagic enterotoxemia and Hemolytic disease** in cattle, sheep, and goats.

☆ *Cl. Perfringens B* produce alpha, beta, and epsilon and cause **Lamb dysentery**.

☆ *Cl. Perfringens C* produce alpha and beta and cause **Goat Enterotoxaemia** and **Struck** in adult sheep, particularly when feed is abundant.

☆ Beta toxin is a necrotizing toxin and initially produces damage to the microvilli with degeneration of mitochondria, with eventual destruction and desquamation of the intestinal epithelial cells and the production of a hemorrhagic enteritis and ulceration of the intestinal mucosa.

☆ *Cl.perfringens E* produce alpha and iota toxin, which is a rare cause of enterotoxaemia in calves and lambs.

☆ *Cl. Perfringens D* produces epsilon toxin. It causes an acute toxemia of ruminants with vascular damage and the damage to nervous system typical of **Pulpy Kidney disease (Overeating Disease)** which is characterized by diarrhea, depression, teeth grinding and convulsions in lambs and young goats and death.

Management and Control

☆ Since the disease is caused by a class of *Cl. perfringens* through toxins produced by the bacteria, it is necessary to observe strict measures while feeding the animals.

☆ Avoid sudden changes in feed.

☆ With the consultation of a veterinarian antibiotic therapy in many instances may be helpful. Mostly long acting penicillin and tetracycline are effective.

☆ Antitoxic serum is one of the choice in acute cases.

☆ Vaccination with multivalent bacterial toxins is very effective way of controlling the disease caused by clostridial species.

☆ Prepartum vaccination of the dam, to provide colostral immunity to the young and subsequent active immunization of the growing animal is recommended for most of the clostridial vaccines.

Important Parasitic Diseases of Livestock

In sheep and goat livestock enterprise, parasitic diseases are common but economically very important. The diseases caused by most of the parasites are not lethal but have potential effect on animal growth, production and reproduction. Sheep are more susceptible to internal parasites than most other types of farm livestock because sheep are close grazers hence more likely to contract parasitic infestation. They are slow to acquire immunity and takes 10 to 12 months for most lambs to develop immunity to parasites. Sheep also suffer a loss of immunity at the time of lambing, which does not restore itself until approximately four weeks after lambing.Their small fecal pellets disintegrate very easily thus releasing the worm larvae onto pastures and heavy stocking rates precipitates the incidence of parasitic diseases. Internal parasitism tend to be much less of a problem under range-type conditions where sheep do not graze the same pasture twice in the same grazing season. They are also less of a problem in arid regions, because parasites require moisture for their development. In a well-managed farm, deworming in the livestock is a routine practice to keep animals healthy and productive. Due to heavy use or long-time use or misuse of anti-parasitic drugs, called "anthelmintics" in the flocks, drug resistance to anthelmintics has increased. The internal parasites that affect sheep and goat are of three classes of *viz.*, Nematodes, Trematodes and Cestodes. Besides these gastrointestinal worms, many protozoan diseases like Babasiosis, theliarais are affecting sheep and goat.

Among the nematodes, the parasite that causes the most problems to sheep and lambs is *Haemonchus contortus.*

☆ Haemonchus is a blood-sucking parasite that pierces the lining of the abomasum ("true" stomach), causing blood plasma and protein loss to the sheep.

☆ The incidence of strongylosis (Haemonchosis) in sheep is above 80 per cent in the Valley.

☆ The disease sometimes become fatal particularly in weaners if not treated in time.

☆ The disease is characterized by anemia, manifested by pale mucous membranes, especially in the lower eye lid, "bottle jaw," an accumulation (swelling) of fluid under the jaw, weight loss with rarely any diarrhea.

Among the trematodes, fluke *Fasciola hepatica* is most frequently found in sheep and cattle and less often in goats and swine.

☆ Acute fascioliasis occurs almost entirely in sheep that causes even death.

☆ Liver flukes require snails as an intermediate host.

☆ The incidence of fasciolosis in sheep varies from 5 to 33 per cent in the Valley.

☆ Adult flukes of Fasciola hepatica are found in the bile ducts and gall bladder. Wandering flukes damage liver tissue and bile ducts in sheep which then become thickened and fibrous.

☆ The eggs are expelled out on the pasture with animal faeces.

☆ Fasciolosisis characterized by weight loss, anaemia, oedema and chronic diarrhea.

☆ Lancet flukes (***Dicrocoelium dendriticum***) in sheep cause little damage to the liver parenchyma except for a moderate to marked thickening of the bile ducts. The incidence of dicrocoeliosis comes to 20 per cent in sheep in the Valley.

Among the cestodes, **Moneizia** is an important tape worm of sheep with its incidence as high as 12 per cent in sheep in the Valley. Tapeworms have an indirect life cycle and require pasture mites to complete their life cycle. Only certain anthelmintics (benzimidazoles) are effective against tapeworms. Although dramatically large numbers of tapeworms may occupy the small intestine, damage to sheep is generally much less than that done by the gastrointestinal nematodes such as Haemonchus and Ostertagia.

Important Protozoan Diseases of Sheep and Goat include Coccidiosis, Babesiosis or Theileriosis

Coccidiosis

It is caused by Coccidia (*Eimeria* spp.) that are single-cell protozoa.

☆ Coccidiosis is very common in sheep, especially young, growing lambs. Older sheep serves as sources of infection for young sheep.

☆ They damage the lining of the small intestine and destroy the crypts.

☆ They are host-specific.

☆ Stress often induces outbreaks of coccidiosis and often follows weaning or shipping stresses.

☆ The incidence of disease is about 70 per cent in lambs, kids and calves in the Valley.

☆ It is characterized by diarrhea (sometimes containing blood or mucous), dehydration, fever, weight loss, loss of appetite, anemia, and death.

☆ Feed additives for the prevention of coccidiosis in lambs are currently in use by the sheep industry. Outbreaks of coccidiosis are usually treated with sulfa drugs and amprolium.

Babesiosis (Piroplasmosis, Texas Fever, Tick Fever)

☆ It is a protozoan parasitic febrile disease of cattle, horses, sheep and swine caused by Babesia species.

☆ In sheep and goats, babesiosis is caused by *Babesia motasi* and *Babesia ovis*. B. ovis usually causes a milder form of the disease than does B. motasi.

☆ The parasite grows and multiplies in the blood corpuscles (erythrocytes) of sheep and goats. Disease is characterized by high fever, anaemia, difficult breathing, loss of appetite, parasitemia and haemoglobinuria (dark redish brown urine) and emaciation.

Toxoplasmosis

☆ Toxoplasmosis is a contagious disease of animals and man caused by protozoon *Toxoplasma gondii*.

☆ It is found most frequently in sheep and is manifested with abortion and stillbirths in ewes. Animals may have fever, generalized tremor and difficult breathing.

Theileriosis

☆ Theileriosis is tick (*Hyalomma* spp.) borne disease of sheep and goats, caused by protozoan species of *Theileria hirci* and *Theileria. ovis*.

☆ *T.hirci* is the cause of an acute and highly fatal disease of sheep and goats.

☆ The subacute and chronic forms have also been reported. Mild infection is noted among young lambs and kids. *Theileria ovis* causes a mild disease in sheep and goats; a disease from which they rapidly recover.

☆ The disease has high morbidity rate of 100 per cent and mortality of 46 – 100 per cent.

☆ The acute form of disease is characterized by high fever (40°C - 41°C), loss of appetite and listlessness, increased heart rate, difficult breathing, edema of the throat, swollen superficial lymph nodes, hyperaemia of the conjunctiva and nasal discharge, emaciation and subsequent death.

Coenurosis (Gid)

☆ It is a disease of brain and spinal cord caused by the intermediate stage of *Taenia multiceps* which inhabits the intestine of dogs, cats and wild carnivores.

☆ Eggs get ingested by sheep from soil or forage soiled by dog faeces. The larvae which reach the brain and spinal cord grow to the *coenurid* stage. Coenurus cerebralis will further mature in the brain and spinal cord.

☆ The clinical disease occurs in sheep that stands intermediate host.

☆ The disease is characterized by blindness, muscular tremor, incoordination, excitability and collapse. Infection with the fully developed larval stage is manifested by salivation, wild expressions, frenzied running and convulsion, deviation of eye and head, loss of function, dullness, incomplete mastication, head pressing and incomplete paralysis.

Echinococcosis (Hydatid Disease)

☆ Hydatid disease occurs in sheep, cattle, swine, horses and humans.

☆ Sheep is an intermediate host and contracts disease by ingesting fodder soiled by dog faeces containing eggs of *Echinococcus granulosus* and *Echinococcus multilocularis*.

☆ These larvae then develop into hydatid cysts in various tissues. The most common sites of cysts are the liver and lungs. The cysts are different sizes and shapes and they contain a clear fluid.

☆ The adult tape worms are found in dogs, cats and other carnivores when they ingest the hydatid cysts containing organs of the intermediate hosts.

Verminous Pneumonia

☆ A disease caused by *Dictyocaulus filaria* which is a common sheep lung worm.

☆ Adult worms live in the bronchi where they lay *eggs* which are coughed up to pharynx and swallowed by the host. The eggs are hatched in the digestive tract and the *larvae* are then expelled in the faeces.

☆ The disease is characterized by difficult breathing, cough and nasal discharge. Fever is noticed when secondary infection is present.

Control and Management of Parasitic Diseases

Although there are different ways of combating parasitism, but each control method in use at present has various limitations. The general opinion is that strategic use of anthelmintics combined with better managemental practices will help in reducing parasitic burdens to considerable levels which in turn will reduce mortality and production losses. For strategic anti-parasitic treatment use of proper drugs at proper dose level and at proper time of the year based on epidemiological studies should be practiced. However, selective deworming of heavily infected animals in a herd after assessing parasitic load may also be employed as and when needed.

The integrated parasitic control includes the following methods

a. Control of parasites and their intermediate hosts by chemicals

    i. Control of parasites in/on animals

    ii. Control of intermediate hosts

b. Control of parasitic stages in environment by adopting better managemental practices

c. Biological control

d. Genetic control

e. Immunological control

f. Molecular control

a. Control of Parasites and their Intermediate Hosts by Chemicals

    i. Chemotherapy and chemoprophylaxis although effective for fighting parasitic diseases, but the use of drugs requires profound knowledge of the biology and epidemiology of the various parasites.

    ii. Forecasting of parasitic infections will help in adopting the curative and prophylactic measures at proper time to prevent outbreaks of disease in already infected animals.

    iii. Treatment of pregnant animals with safe anthelmintic is recommended and there is no reason not to administer anthelmintics in pregnant or recently partured animals that probably is the major reason that such animals fall prey to parasitic diseases. Pregnant and recently parturated animals are more susceptible to parasitic infections due to temporary relaxation in their immunity (peri- parturient and post-parturient rise in faecal egg counts), hence these animals should be treated with safer anthelmintics. Treatment of gastrointestinal nematodes in pregnant animals with fenbedazole instead of albendazole is safer and has a similar spectrum of activity.

    iv. Similarly larval stages of certain nematodes *e.g.*, *Haemonchus* and *Oestertagia* undergo arrested development (hypobiosis) within the body of host at the time when environmental conditions are not safer for their development and survival (winter in Kashmir). Resumption of development of these arrested larvae upon return of favourable conditions which is technically called as spring rise phenomenon plays an important role in survival of these nematodes. Therefore, anthelmintic treatment of animals for haemonchosis in spring (March) will help in controlling these infections to a greater extent by reducing contamination of grazing land.

There are two main groups of drugs used for treatment of trematode and cestode infections in domestic animals. These are phenol derivatives including salicylanides (niclosamide, cliozanide, nitroxynil, diamfenitide) and benzimidazoles(albendazole, fenbendazole, luxabendazole, triclabendazole).

However all is not good with anthelmintics, there is development of drug resistance, risk of drug residues in meat and milk. The pre-slaughter withdrawal period of flukicides varies from 14 days (oxycloxanide) to 33 days (nitroxynil). Similarly the milk of cows which have been treated with albendazole, oxycloxanide and nitroxynil should not be used for 4 to 5 days.

Control of Intermediate Hosts by Chemicals

    i. Snails which act as intermediate hosts of flukes can be effectively controlled by use of molluscides like copper sulphate or N-tritylomorpholine. Molluscides should be applied in spring or and summer. Spring applications are easy to apply, highly effective, killing off over wintered infected snails and parent snails which would supply the nucleus of the years breeding population. Mid-summer applications are not always as effective as spring applications

ii. In ponds the copper sulphate should be added in such a way so that total concentration becomes 1:50000 to 1: 100000

b. Control of Parasitic Stages in Environment by Adopting better Managemental Practices

i. Proper disposal of animal excreta: Manure must be regularly and frequently removed from animal houses and spread on fields directly in thin layer or stacked in large compact heaps. If the manure is stacked in large compact heaps, it ferments and the heat thus produced kills the eggs and larvae of most of the internal parasites.

ii. Preventing animals from grazing in marshy areas.

iii. Alternate grazing of pasture/grazing lands with hosts of different species.

iv. Alternate grazing with hosts of same species (younger animals first and older animals latter).

v. Pasture resting if possible (six months under moist and temperate conditions and two months under hot and arid conditions).

vi. Pasture burning: If the pasture is heavily infected with larvae of strongyle worms or seed ticks it can be burnt to control infections with these worms Ploughing and reseeding of infected pasture/grazing land.

c. Biological Control

Biological control means control of any harmful pest by using its natural enemies. In nature every species has got a set of natural enemies and their use can be exploited for keeping the population of species in question under control.

i. For control of ticks certain hymenoptercan insects like *Hunterellus* spp. and *Ixodiphagus* spp. are used.

ii. For biological control of mosquitoes we can use larviparous fishes and certain water plants. Similarly scientists are trying to isolate pathogens of mosquitoes like bacteria, viruses *etc.* which can be grown in the laboratory and introduced in breeding places of mosquitoes to create epidemics in mosquitoes.

iii. Biological control of gastrointestinal nematodes involving nematode destroying fungi is a new concept. The nematode destroying fungi occupy different niches in the soil where they feed on variety of free living soil nematodes or plant parasitic nematodes or decaying organic matter. A large proportion of nematophagous fungi known today are assigned to the class-deoteromycotina.

d. Genetic Control

i. Genetic control means use of any condition or treatment that can reduce the reproductive potential of noxious agent by altering or replacing their genetic material. This can be done by sterile mating and interbreeding of incompatible strains. These two methods have been used for control of mosquitoes under experimental conditions.

ii. The eradication of screw worm fly *Cochliomyia* (*Callitroga*) *homnivorax* from USA by release of male flies sterilized by irradiation has been a great success. The fly was eradicated from the island of Curacao and shore of Florida with outstanding success.

e. Immunological Control

There are very few commercial vaccinesavailable for control of parasitic diseases. These are either live or dead vaccines *e.g.*, **Dictol-** against *Dictyocaulus viviparous*, **Rakshavac-T**-against *Theileria annulata* **Coccivac** and **Immunocox** against poultry coccidiosis.

f. Molecular Control

In molecular control method naked DNA fragment coding for a protective antigen itself is introduced into the body. Following introduction into body, various tissues including muscles, or lymphoid tissue can uptake the naked DNA and express the foreign gene products which are then presented to antigen processing cells for generating strong cell mediated and humoral immune response. The nucleic acid sequences or the whole gene could be introduced via a viral vector such as vaccinia, carpipox, swine pox or via a plasmid. The introduction of naked nucleic acid *in vivo* via a vector for purpose of generating immune response is called naked DNA vaccine

Naked DNA vaccines have been produced and experimentally used against various protozoan parasites like, *Leishmania major*, *Theleria annulata*, *Toxoplasma gondii*, *Plasmodium* spp., *Eimeria* spp. *etc.*

Fecal Egg Analysis

Fecal egg analysis is an important part of an internal parasite control program. Primarily, a fecal analysis tells you how contaminated your pastures are. Fecal analysis can also be used to make selection and culling decisions by identifying animals with both high and low egg counts. The most valuable use of fecal egg analysis is to determine drug resistance.

The test to determine drug resistance is called the fecal egg count reduction test (FECRT). In FECRT, animal are weighed and dewormed with the test anthelmintic. Fecal samples are collected twice, first at the time of deworming and second, 7 to 14 days later. Ideally 10 animals should be tested for each anthelmintic. Fecal samples should also be collected and analyzed for a similar group of untreated animals. Effective anthelmintic should reduce fecal egg counts by 90 percent. There is severe drug resistance if treatment fails to reduce egg counts by more than 60 percent.

Since fecal counts only estimate the parasite load, there is no clear cut level at which deworming is indicated. As a general guide, a level of about 500 eggs per gram of feces would indicate that deworming is needed for sheep. Liver flukes are prolific egg producers, but egg counts are not necessarily a good indication of infection levels. Coccidia eggs are very small, than a Strongyle egg as such oocysts in faeces are only a moderate indicator of level of infection.

The FAMACHA© system was developed in South Africa due to the emergence of drug-resistant worms. The system utilizes an eye anemia guide to evaluate the eyelid color of a sheep (or goat) to determine the severity of parasite infection (as evidenced by anemia) and the need for deworming. A bright red color indicates that the animal has few or no worms or that the sheep has the capacity to tolerate its worms. An almost white eyelid color a warning sign of very bad anemia; the worms present in the sheep's gut are in such numbers they are draining the animal of blood. If left untreated, such an animal will soon die.The FAMACHA© chart contains five eye scores (1-5), which have been correlated with packed cell volumes. Animals in categories 1 (PCV ≥ 28, red) or 2 (PCV-23-27, red-pink) do not require treatment whereas animals in categories 4 (PCV 13-17, pink whilte) and 5 (PCV ≤ 12, white) do require treatment whereas animals in category 3 (PCV 18-22, Pink) may or may not require treatment depending upon other factors. The employment of FAMACHA system will result into few animals being treated thus slashing down drug resistance.

Chapter 7

Important Breeds of Sheep and Goats

Sheep and goats provide nutritional security and supplementary income to the poor small or marginal farmers in rural India. In most of the rural setups, sheep and goat are kept along with cattle and poultry in an integrated agriculture system. Sheep and goat rearing is preferred over cattle because of its low capital investment and simple housing and feeding. There are several sheep and goat breeds adapted to particular agro-climatic conditions in India. Most of sheep are dual purpose providing mutton as well as wool whereas most of goats are dairy goats. The breeds of sheep and their main product in parenthesis of different agro-ecological zones of India are given here under.

North Temperate	North-Western Arid and Semi Arid	Southern Peninsular	Eastern
Bhakarwal (CW)	Chokla (CW)	Bellary (MCW)	Balangir (MCW)
Changthangi (CW)	Hissardale (AW)	Coimbatore (MCW)	Bonpala (MCW)
Gaddi (CW)	Jaisalmeri (MCW)	Daccani (M)	Chottanagpuri
Gurez (CW)	Jalauni (MCW)	Hassan (M)	(MCW)
Karnah (AW)	Kheri (MCW)	Kanguri (M)	Ganjam (MCW)
Kashmir Merino (AW)	Magra (CW)	Kilakarsal (M)	Garole (M)
Poonchi (CW)	Malpura (MCW)	Madras Red (M)	Tibetan (CW)
Rampur Bushair (CW)	Marwari (MCW)	Mandya (M)	
	Muzaffarnagari	Mecheri (M)	
	(MCW)	Nellore (M)	
	Nali (CW)	Nilgiri (AW)	
	Patanwadi (CW)	Rammand White (M)	
	Pugal (MCW)	Tiruchy Black (M)	
	Sonadi (MCW)	Vembur (M)	
	Munjal (M)		

(AW)- Apparel wool; (CW)-Carpet wool; (MCW)- Mutton and Carpet wool; (M)-Mutton.

Details of some of the Important Breeds of Sheep

BAKERWALI

The animal is reared by nomadic tribes called Bakerwals and is migratory sheep.

☆ Animals get migrated during summer to alpine and subalpine pastures of Kashmir Valley or low lying hills of Jammu and during winter to subtropics of Jammu and Punjab State.

☆ Being migratory these sheep live in open throughout the year.

☆ These sheep are hardy and sturdy and are excellent climbers in-spite of its big bulk.

☆ The males are generally horned and ewes hornless.

☆ Some flocks are fat tailed.

☆ Ears are generally long, broad and dropping.

☆ These sheep grow coloured coarse wool, which is used locally for manufacture of coarse lohis (Small blankets).

☆ Wool yield reaches 1.6 kg per annum per animal.

BALANGIRI

☆ It is spread over north western districts of Orissa, Balangir, Sambalpur and Sundargarh.

☆ They are medium sized, having white or light brown or of mixed colour.

☆ The ears are small and stumpy.

☆ Males are horned and females are polled.

☆ Fleece is extremely coarse, hairy and open.

☆ Adult body of male averages 24 kg and that of female 18 kgs.

BHARAT MERINO SHEEP

☆ Bharat Merino sheep developed by crossbreeding indigenous Chokla and Nali sheep with Rambouillet and Merino rams and stabilised at 75 per cent exotic inheritance.

☆ It has the potential as an import substitute for exotic fine wool inheritance.

☆ The annual greasy wool production is 2.5 kg with fibre diameter of 19-20 microns, medullation less than one percent and staple length of 78 cm.

☆ Bharat Merino sheep were distributed to Kolar District of Karnataka and in Sathyamangalam and Thalavadi areas of Erode District in Tamilnadu.

☆ The average body weight of Bharat Merino sheep at Kolar District was found to be 45 kg and 32 kg, ranged from 38-70 kg and 28-40 kg for adult male and female respectively.

☆ Birth weight of lamb was 4.0 kg with range of 3.5-4.5 kg. The weight at 3, 6, and 12 months were 18, 25 and 30 kg, respectively.

CHANGTHANGI

- ☆ Changthangi sheep are found in Changthang Sub-Division of Leh District of J&K State.
- ☆ It is locally known as changluk.
- ☆ It is seasonal breeder with breeding season from July to December.
- ☆ Animals are big sized, usually coloured.
- ☆ Wool is coarse, long and yield averages to 1.5 kg per annum per animal.
- ☆ Sheep are used as a transport animal in the mountains.
- ☆ The average body weight in male is 30kgs and of female 25kg.

CHOKLA

- ☆ This breed is distributed in Churu, Jhunjhunu, Sikarand bordering areas of Bikaner, Jaipur and Nagaur districts of Rajasthan.
- ☆ The animals are light to medium sized. The face, generally devoid of wool, is reddish brown or dark brown, and the colour may extend up to the middle of the neck.
- ☆ The ears are small to medium in length and tubular.
- ☆ The coat is dense and relatively fine, covering the entire body including the belly and the greater part of the legs.
- ☆ Chokla is fine carpet wool Indian sheep and reared basically for its wool quality and suitability for migration.
- ☆ Chokla grows the finest carpet wool of all the Indian breeds ranging from 54s to 60s count. The wool produced by Chokla sheep is heterogeneous and is generally mixed with coarser fleece of other sheep before utilization as carpet wool.
- ☆ Chokla produces wool with average fiber diameter and medullation percentage of around 30microns and 30 per cent with staple length of more than 6.0 cm suitable for all kind of carpet preparation.
- ☆ Since 1992, through intensive selection and improved management, six month weight of the sheep has increased significantly from 16.51 kg to 24.83 kg.

CHOTTANAGPURI

- ☆ This breed is distributed in Chottanagpur, Ranchi, Palamau, Hazaribagh, Singhbhum, Dhanbad and Santhal Parganas of Jharkhand, and Bankura district of West Bengal.
- ☆ Animals are small, light in weight with light grey and brown colour.
- ☆ Ears are small and parallel to the head.
- ☆ Fleece is coarse, hairy and open and is generally not clipped.

COIMBATORE

☆ It is distributed in Coimbatore district and adjoining Dindigul district of Tamil Nadu.

☆ Medium-sized animals, white with black or brown spots.

☆ Ears are medium-sized and directed outward and backward.

☆ Fleece is white, coarse, hairy and open.

☆ Rams are both horned and polled while ewes are hornless.

☆ Average body weights at birth, three, six and twelve months of age are 2.16, 7.50, 10.83 and 14.77 kg, respectively.

☆ Adult male body weight averages 25 kg and female 20 kg.

DECCANI

☆ The Deccani breed of sheep is widely distributed in the Deccan plateau across the three states of Maharashtra, Andhra Pradesh and Karnataka.

☆ The breed has a thin neck, narrow chest, prominent spinal processes.

☆ It has Roman nose and dropping ears.

☆ The colour is dominantly black, with some grey and roan.

☆ Average body weights at birth, three, six, nine and twelve months of age are 3.13, 14.30, 18.20, 20.10 and 22.57 kg, respectively.

☆ Average weaning weight of the Deccani is 13.23 kg and final weight at six months of age reaches 22.65 kg.

☆ Deccani has the great potential for mutton production under intensive system of management and are maintained chiefly for mutton.

GADDI OR BHADARWAHI

☆ Gaddi sheep are distributed in Kistwar and Bhadarwah,Ramnagar, Udampur in Jammu province of Jammu and Kashmir. It is also found in Kullu and Kangra valleys of Himachal Pradesh,Nainital, Tehri Garhwal and Chamoli districts of Uttar Pradesh.

☆ The animals are medium sized, usually white. Although tan, brown and black and their mixtures are also seen.

☆ Males are horned and females are largely polled, however, 10 to 15 per cent females are also horned.

☆ Wool is fine and lustrous; average annual yield is 1.13 kg per sheep, clipped thrice a year.

☆ Means of birth weight at 3, 6, 9 and 12 months weight of lambs are 2.22, 7.64, 11.01, 14.01 and 16.19 kg, respectively under farm conditions.

☆ Adult body weight varies from 30 to 34 kgs.

☆ Wool yield varies from 500g to 700g with fiber diameter of 29 microns and medullation percentage of 26.

GAROLE

☆ Sheep are reputed for multiple births and are found in the Sunderban area of West Bengal.

☆ These sheep are reported to have contributed prolificacy to the Booroola Merino sheep.

☆ Garole Wool is for rough carpet use. The average fibre diameter, medullation, staple length and crimp/cm. are 67.82 µ, 75.17 per cent, 5.09 cm and 2.08 respectively.

☆ Litter size at first lambing is two and at subsequent lambing is 2 to 3. Prolificacy reported is single 25-30 per cent, twin 55-60 per cent, triplet 15-20 per cent and quadruplet 12 per cent.

GUREZI

☆ It is inhabitant of Gurez tehsil of Kashmir Valley

☆ It is the biggest among the Kashmiri sheep breeds.

☆ Coat colour is white with coarse wool.

☆ They have short ears and are polled predominantly.

☆ Wool yield is about 1.25 to 1.5 Kg per year per animal.

☆ Adult body weight varies from 36 kgs to 41kgs.

KARNAHI

☆ It is inhabitant of Karnah Tehsil of Kashmir, at an attitude of 1200-4600 meters.

☆ The animals are robust, having long face and a prominent nose.

☆ Rams have big curved horns.

☆ The fleece is relatively fine though shorter than that of Guresi, breed of sheep.

☆ Wool yield reaches to 1 Kg to 1.25kg per annum per animal. Wool is fine with average fiber diameter of 29.70 µ (micron) and staple length of 9.36 centimeters.

☆ Adult body weight varies from 31 to 38kgs.

HASSAN

☆ Distributed in Hassan district of Karnataka.

☆ Small sized animals, having white body with light brown or black spots.

☆ Ears are medium-long and drooping; ear length.

☆ Majority of males are horned and females are usually polled.

☆ Fleece is white, extremely coarse and open; legs and belly are generally devoid of wool.

☆ This breed is very hardy and capable to travel long distances.

HISSARDALE

- ☆ Hissardale was evolved at the Government Livestock Farm, Hissar, through crossbreeding Australian Merino rams with Bikaneri (Magra) ewes and stabilizing the exotic inheritance at about 75 per cent.

- ☆ There is a small flock of this breed at the Government Livestock Farm, Hissar.

- ☆ The rams of this breed were earlier distributed in the hilly regions of Kullu, Kangra *etc.*

JAISALMERI

- ☆ Jaisalmeri breed is found in Jaisalmer, Banner and Jodhpur districts of Rajasthan.

- ☆ The animals are tall and wellbuilt with black or dark brown face and the colour extending up to the neck and typical Roman nose.

- ☆ Long drooping ears, generally with a cartilaginous appendage are seen.

- ☆ Both sexes are polled.

- ☆ The tail is medium to long.

- ☆ The fleece colour is white and is of medium carpet quality and not very dense.

KASHMIR MERINO

- ☆ This breed originated from crosses of different Merino types with predominantly migratory native sheep breeds such as Gaddi, Bhakarwal and Poonchi.

- ☆ Local Kashmir valley ewes were crossed with Australian Merino Rams and F1 Ewes were bred to Delain Rams of USA. F_2 were bred among themselves after proper selection on the basis of wool quality and body weight. The matting among F_2 generation continued till a breed with steady and uniform characters evolved which was named as Kashmir Merino.

- ☆ The level of inheritance varies from very low to almost 100 per cent Merino, though a level from 50 to 75 per cent predominates.

- ☆ The adult rams weighs from 54-60 kg and ewe from 45-50 kg.

- ☆ The fleece weigh ranges from 3-4 kgs.

- ☆ The breed is comparable to some of the finest wool breeds of the world with fibre diameter of 20-24 Microns.

KENDRAPADA

- ☆ This sheep is identified as another prolific sheep of India after Garole of West Bengal which carry *FecB* mutation.

- ☆ Kendrapada is distributed in Bhadrak, Konark and Puri district of coastal area of Orissa.

☆ Kendrapada is an excellent medium stature meat type sheep. The adult body weight of sheep was about 23 kg.

☆ The coat colour varies from white to dark brown. Some black animals and black/white spot on body are also found.

KENGURI

☆ Distribution is hilly tracts of Raichur district (particularly Lingasagar, Sethanaur and Gangarati taluks) of Karnataka. The breed is also known as Tenguri.

☆ Medium-sized animals.

☆ The body coat is dark brown or of coconut colour.

☆ Some Kenguri sheep have black belly and are known as Jodka. A few sheep, known as Masaka, are a mixture of brown and black colour.

☆ Ears are medium long and drooping.

☆ Males are horned; females are generally polled.

☆ Kenguri sheep are maintained for mutton.

KHERI

☆ Kheri sheep evolved in the farmers flock under the field conditions especially in the areas that are important for sheep migration in Rajasthan.

☆ The animals of this breed have established owing to their ability to walk long distances and ability to survive on limited amount of coarse feed.

☆ The animals of this breed can sustain stress and on return of favorable condition, regain faster resulting in better reproduction rate and growth of lambs as compared to prevalent breeds in the area.

☆ Birth, 3, 6 month weight in Kheri are 2.97±0.05, 14.76±0.22 and 17.49±0.29 kg respectively

KILAKARSAL

☆ Distributed in Ramnathpuram, Madurai, Thanjavur and Ramnad districts of Tamil Nadu.

☆ It is a medium-sized animal.

☆ Coat is dark tan, with black spots on head (particularly the eyelids and lower jaw), belly and legs.

☆ Ears are medium sized.

☆ Tail is small and thin.

☆ Males have thick twisted horns.

☆ Most animals have wattles.

☆ Average body weights at birth, three, six and twelve months of age are 2.29, 8.53, 14.15 and 27.26 Kg, respectively.

MADRAS RED

☆ Distributed in Chennai, Kancheepuram, Tiruvellore, Villupuram and adjoining areas of Vellore, Cuddalore and Thiruvannamalai districts of Tamil Nadu.

☆ Medium-sized animals.

☆ Body colour is predominantly brown, the intensity varying from light tan to dark brown; some animals have white markings on the forehead, inside the thighs and on the lower abdomen.

☆ Ears are medium long and drooping.

☆ Tail is short and thin.

☆ Rams have strong corrugated and twisted horns; the ewes are polled.

☆ The body is covered with short hairs which are not shorn.

☆ Average body weights at birth, three, six and twelve months of age are 2.71, 9.97, 14.84 and 21.03 kg, respectively. Adult male weighs 36 kgs and female 24 kgs.

☆ Dressing percentage is around 49.

MAGRA

☆ Magra sheep is distributed in Bikaner, Nagaur, Jaisalmer and Churu districts of Rajasthan. However, animals true to the breed type are found only in the eastern and southern parts of Bikaner district.

☆ The animals are medium to large in size.

☆ White face with light brown patches around the eyes is characteristic of this breed.

☆ Skin colour is pink Ears are small to medium and tubular.

☆ Both sexes are polled. Tail is medium in length and thin.

☆ Fleece is of medium carpet quality, extremely white and lustrous and not very dense. Fibre diameter ranged between 32.5 to 38μ with staple length from 4.2 to 6.8cm

☆ Average body weights at birth, six and twelve months of age are 3.04, 20.64 and 29.23 Kg, respectively under field conditions.

MAIPURA

☆ Malpura sheep are found in Jaipur, Tonk, Sawaimadhopur and adjacent areas of Ajmer, Bhilwara and Bundi districts in Rajasthan.

☆ The animals are fairly wellbuilt, with long legs.

☆ Face is light brown. Ears are short and tubular, with a small cartilaginous appendage on the upper side.

☆ Both sexes are polled.

☆ Tail is medium to long and thin.

☆ The fleece is white, extremely coarse and hairy.

☆ Means of birth, 3, 6 and 12 month's weight of lambs are 3.02, 15.41, 20.80 and 25.60 kg, respectively under farm conditions.

☆ The average fibre diameter is 41.67μ with medullation of 75.9 per cent and staple length 4.9cm.

MANDYA

☆ It is also known as Bannur and Bandur,distributed in Mandya district and bordering Mysore district of Karnataka.

☆ Relatively small animals but compact body with a typical reversed U-shape conformation from the rear.

☆ Colour is white, but in some cases face is light brown, and this colour may extend to the neck.

☆ Ears are long, leafy and drooping. Slightly Roman nose.

☆ Tail is short and thin. A large percentage of animals carry wattles.

☆ Both sexes are polled.

☆ Coat is extremely coarse and hairy.

☆ Evenly placed short and stumpy legs and wide apart hipbones indicated best mutton type conformation of the breed among the Indian breeds.

☆ Average body weights at birth, three, six and twelve months of age are 2.02, 9.44, 14.61 and 21.34 kg, respectively.

MARWARI

☆ Marwari sheep are distributed in Jodhpur, Jalore, Nagaur, Pali and Barmer districts extending up to Ajmer and Udaipur districts of Rajasthan and the Jeoria region of Gujarat.

☆ The animals are medium size with black face, the colour extending to the lower part of neck.

☆ Ears are extremely small and tubular. Wattles are often present

☆ Both sexes are polled.

☆ Tail is short to medium and thin.

☆ The fleece is white and not very dense.

☆ Means of body weight at birth, 3, 6, 9 and 12 month's of lambs are 3.05, 14.74, 19.33, 22.85 and 25.90 kg, respectively under farm conditions.

☆ The yield of wool per year is 0.90-1.81 kg per animal. Average fibre diameter, medullation and staple length are 31.9μ, 50.8 per cent and 5.35cm respectively.

MECHERI

☆ Distributed in Mecheri, Kolathoor, Nangavalli, Omalur and Tarmangalam Panchayat Union areas of Salem district and Bhavani taluk of Coimbatore district of Tamil Nadu.

☆ Medium-sized animals, and light brown in colour.

☆ Both the sexes are polled.

☆ Body is covered with very short hairs which are not shorn.

☆ The skin is of the highest quality of sheep breeds in India and is highly prized.

☆ Average body weights at birth, three, six, nine and twelve months of age are 2.23, 10.07, 13.73, 18.62 and 21.12 for male lambs and corresponding value for female lambs are 2.28, 9.70, 13.53, 15.84 and 18.02 kg, respectively under farm conditions. Adult male weighs 36 kgs and female 22 kgs.

MUZZAFARNAGRI

☆ This breed is distributed in Muzzafarnagar, Bulandshaher, Sahranpur, Meerut, bijnor andDehradun districts of Uttar Pradesh and parts of Delhi and Haryana.

☆ The animals are medium to large in size. Face line is slightly convex.

☆ Ears and face are occasionally black. Ears are long and drooping.

☆ Both sexes are polled. Males occasionally show rudimentary horns.

☆ Tail is extremely long and reaches fetlock.

☆ The fleece is white, coarse and open. Belly and legs are devoid of wool.

☆ Means for lambs 1st and 2nd six monthly and adult annual clips are 582.17, 538.75 and 1217.62g, respectively under farm conditions.

☆ The overall averages body weights are 3.63, 15.59, 23.52, 27.14 and 30.76kg, respectively at birth, 3, 6, 9 and 12 month age.

☆ Means of wool quality attributes *viz*. fibre diameter, hetrofibres, hairy fibres, medullation and staple length are 38.39±1.36μ, 14.35±1.37 per cent, 46.89±3.42 per cent, 61.03±4.33 per cent and 5.09±0.30cm, respectively.

NALI

☆ The Nali sheep is found in Ganganagar, Churu and Jhunjhunu districts of Rajasthan, southern part of Hissar and Rotak districts of Haryana.

☆ The animals are medium sized.

☆ Face colour is light brown and skin colour is pink. Fleece is white, coarse, dense and long stapled.

☆ Both sexes are polled.

☆ Ears are large and leafy. Tail is short to medium and thin.

☆ Means of weight at birth, 3, 6, 9 and 12 months of lambs are 2.43, 10.74, 14.93, 17.13 and 19.64 kg, respectively under farm conditions.

☆ Average fibre diameter, medullation and staple length are 29.89μ, 41.14 per cent and 6.79cm respectively.

NELLORE

☆ Distributed in Nellore district and neighbouring areas of Prakasham and Ongole districts of Andhra Pradesh.

☆ Three varieties are distinguished, primarily on the basis of colour: "Palla", completely white "Jodipi", white with black spots, particularly around the lips, eyes and lower jaw and "Dora", completely brown.

☆ Relatively tall animals with little hair except at brisket, withers and breech.

☆ The rams are horned and ewes are almost always polled.

☆ The ears are long and drooping and most of the animals carry wattles.

☆ The overall averages of body weight of Nellore sheep are 2.95, 13.91, 17.38, 22.39 and 26.61 kg at birth, 3, 6, 9 and 12 month age respectively.

PATANWADI

☆ Patanwadi is also called desi, Kutchi, Vadhiyari and Charotari.

☆ The animals, in general, are medium to large with relatively long legs.

☆ They have typical Roman nose with brown face which may be tan in a few cases.

☆ Ears are medium to large, tubular with a hairy tuft.

☆ The tail is thin and short.

☆ Both sexes are polled.

☆ Means of weight at birth, 3, 6, 9 and 12 months of lambs are 3.23, 14.26, 17.67, 20.76 and 24.22 kg, respectively under farm conditions.

☆ Average fibre diameter and medullation are 29.11μ and 38.41 per cent respectively.

POONCHI

☆ This breed of sheep is found in Poonch and surrounding places situated at a high elevation in J&K State.

☆ Animals are long sized.

☆ Mostly hornless with short tail which is thick at the base.

☆ Ears are generally short.

☆ Coat colour is predominantly white.

☆ These sheep are best for wool production and are raised on rich summer pastures and are stall fed during winter on stored grasses and fodders.

☆ Wool yield averages 1.6 kg per annum which is medium fine with average fiber diameter of 32 microns.

RAMANADHAPURAM WHITE

☆ This is distributed in Ramanadhapuram, Sivagangai, and Virudhunagar districts of Tamilnadu.

★ It is meat purpose breed.

★ It has medium sized body.

★ Majority of them are white in color.

★ Certain goats hold black colored stripes all over their body.

★ Adult males have their bent horns, whereas females with absence of horns.

★ Legs are smaller and slender.

★ Adult male average body weight reaches 31kg and female 23kg.

SANDYNO

★ Sandyno breed was developed by crossing Nilagiri sheep with Merino and Rambouillet. The breed has ¾ inheritance from Nilagiri and 5/8 inheritance from Merino/Rambouillet breeds.

★ The breed has been field tested and found to adapt well to the local climatic and environmental conditions.

★ The Sandyno sheep grow to a body weight of 24 kg in males and 20 kg in females at yearling stage.

★ The average wool yield is 2.2 kg.

SHAHABADI

★ Shahabadi is found in Shahabad, Patna and Gaya districts of Bihar/ Jharkhand state.

★ The animals are of medium size and leggy.

★ The fleece is mostly grey and sometimes with black spots.

★ The ears are of medium size and drooping.

★ The tail is extremely long and thin.

★ Both sexes are polled.

★ Fleece is extremely coarse, hairy and open.

★ Average six monthly greasy fleece yield is 240 g. Fibre diameter is 49.83 µ with Medullation percent of 87.08.

SONADI

★ Sonadi is found in Udaipur and Dungarpur districts and, to some extent, Chittorgarh district of Rajasthan and also extends to northern Gujarat.

★ The Animals are fairly well built, somewhat smaller than Malpura, with long legs.

★ Light brown face with the colour extending to the middle of the neck.

★ Ears are large, flat and drooping; Ears generally have a cartilaginous appendage.

★ Tail is long and thin.

★ The fleece is white, extremely coarse and hairy.

☆ Means of weight at birth, 3, 6, 9 and 12 months of lambs are 2.52, 10.78, 14.98, 17.32 and 21.76 kg, respectively under farm conditions.

TIBETAN

☆ The Tibetan breed is found in northern Sikkim and Kameng district of Arunachal Pradesh.

☆ Animals are medium sized, mostly white with black or brown face; brown and white spots are also found on the body.

☆ Both the sexes are horned.

☆ The nose is convex, giving a typical Roman nose.

☆ The ears are small, broad and drooping.

☆ The fleece is relatively fine and dense.

☆ Average six monthly greasy fleece yield ranges between 400-900 g Staple length is 7.24 cm, Fibre diameter is 19.3 µ with Medullation percent of 13.22.

TIRUCHY BLACK

☆ Distributed in Perambalur, Ariyalur and Tiruchy, Kallakurichy taluk of South- Arcot district, Viraganur area of Attur taluk of Salem district, Tirupathur and Tiruvannamalai taluks of North Arcot district of Tamil Nadu.

☆ Males are horned and ewes are polled.

☆ Ears are short and directed downward and forward.

☆ Tail is short and thin.

☆ The fleece is extremely coarse, hairy and open.

☆ Average body weights at birth, three, six and twelve months of age are 2.13, 9.46, 10.73 and 16.80 Kg, respectively.

☆ Adult male body weight averages 26kg and female 19kg.

VEMBUR

☆ It is distributed in Vembur, melakarandhai, keezhakarandhai, nagalapuram regions, Tuticorin and Virudhunagar districts of Tamilnadu.

☆ It is meat purpose breed.

☆ These are taller breeds.

☆ They have white color skin with red color spots over their body.

☆ Ears are drooped out.

☆ Tail is smaller and slender.

☆ Adult males are found with horns and absence of horns in case of females.

☆ Adult male average body weight reaches 35kgs and females 28kgs.

Some of Important Exotic Sheep Breeds

CHEVIOT

☆ Is a medium wool breed, primarily developed in Scotland.

☆ The breed is small with erect ears, a clean white face and white legs, covered with short white hair.

☆ The nose, lips and feet are black.

☆ Rams weigh on an average upto 80 kg and ewes up to 55kg.

CORRIEDALE

☆ The Corriedale was developed in New Zealand and Australia during the late 1800s' from crossing Lincoln or Leicester rams with Merino females. Similar crosses were also being developed in Australia during this time.

☆ The breed is now distributed worldwide, making up the greatest population of all sheep in South America and thrives throughout Asia, North America and South Africa.

☆ Its popularity now suggests it is the second most significant breed in the world after Merinos.

☆ The Corriedale is a dual-purpose sheep.

☆ It is large-framed, polled with good carcass quality. Mature rams weigh from 175 to 275 pounds (79-125 kg) and ewes from 130 to 180 pounds (59-81 kg).

☆ The Corriedale produces bulky, high-yielding wool from 10 to 17 pounds (4.5-7.7 kg). The fibre diameter ranging from 31.5 to 24.5 micron.

DORPER SHEEP

☆ Dorper belongs to arid climatic condition, this breed has the ability to adjust to varying seasonal changes.

☆ It is highly popular in western regions.

☆ The body has a good combination of hair and wool.

☆ They vary from medium to large size and produces delicious mutton.

DORSET

☆ It has evolved from Merino sheep crossed with the horned sheep of Wales, in Southwest England that spread over Dorset, Somerset, Devon, and most of Wales and were called Horned Dorsets.

☆ Polled Dorsets originated at North Carolina State College, Raleigh, NC, and were apparently the result of a mutation which occurred in the pure bred Horned Dorset flock at the college.

☆ Both horned and polled Dorsets are all-white sheep of medium size having good body length and muscle conformation to produce delicious meat.

☆ It is a hardy breed and capable of performing well under most conditions.

☆ The sheep has an amazing milk producing and meat giving ability.

☆ This is among the most popular white face sheep in the world and has a huge presence all over the globe.

☆ Dorset rams weigh from 225 to 275 pounds and ewes from 150 to 200 pounds at maturity.

☆ Dorset fleeces average five to nine pounds (2.25-4 kg) in the ewes. The fibre diameter ranges from 33.0 to 27.0 microns.

☆ Their numbers make them the second largest breed in total numbers in the USA, ranking below only the Suffolk breed.

FEC- B SHEEP

☆ Originated in Australia by crossing the pre-existing Merino flock with Booroola Sheep, originally imported from West Bengal (Garolle) India.

☆ Have a dominant allele known as Fec-B, a gene that produces multiple births by increasing rate of ovulation

☆ Regularly produce twins and some triplets.

☆ Mature ram weighs from 38-42 kg and ewe from 30- 35 kg.

☆ Typically small sized with white face which is free of dark fibers.

☆ Potential means of genetically improving the reproductive component of productivity.

HAMPSHIRE SHEEP

☆ It is known for its excellent and delicious mutton.

☆ It is dark faced and hornless breed.This breed is a result of cross culture, and that is the reason for its varying skin tone.

☆ They are medium sized, quickly growing breed.

☆ The sheep has medium wool.

LINCOLN SHEEP

☆ This sheep remains popular worldwide and weights between 260 to 350 pounds.

☆ It is popular for its lovely and finest wool and fleece, which is demanded all over the world for weaving and designing.

MERINO

☆ The most popular fine wool breed of the world, originated in Spain.

☆ It is a white faced sheep with white feet.

☆ Rams have horns whereas the ewes are hornless.

☆ Most of the head and legs are covered by wool.

☆ The ewes live and yield longer than any other breed

☆ The animal is extremely hardy being able to survive under adverse weather and poor grazing conditions.

RAMBOUILLET

☆ It was developed in France.

☆ This breed has a large head with white hair around the nose and ears.

☆ Rams have horns and ewes are hornless.

☆ Rams weigh as much as 125 kg and ewes up to a maximum of 90 kg.

☆ It produces an excellent fine-wool fleece.

☆ The fleece is heavy, close, compact, covering most of the body including face and legs.

SOUTHDOWN

☆ The Southdown were developed in Sussex, England during the late 1700 and early 1800s'.

☆ The Southdown is best suited for farm flock production.

☆ It is a medium to small sized breed with a gray to mouse-brown face and lower legs and is polled (hornless).

☆ Southdown are an early maturing breed with good lambing ability and average milk production.

☆ Southdown rams weigh from 190 to 230 pounds (86-104 kg) and ewes from 130 to 180 pounds (59-81 kg) at maturity.

☆ Fleece weights from mature ewe are between five and eight pounds (2.25-3.6 kg). The fleeces are considered medium wool type with a fibre diameter of 23.5 to 29.0 microns.

SUFFOLK SHEEP

☆ It is native of U.K. and is large animal with black face, ears and legs.

☆ Head and ears entirely free from wool.

☆ Both rams and ewes are polled though rams sometimes have scars.

☆ Its average wool yield 2-3 kg.

☆ Mature Rams weigh 100-135 kg and ewes from 70-100 kg.

☆ Ewes are very prolific and excellent milkers.

☆ This is among the largest rowing breed, which offers tasty mutton.

Some of Important Goat Breeds

BAKERWAL

☆ Bakerwal is derived from the Gojri/Urdu/Punjabi/Kashmiri/Dogri terms, *bakra* meaning goat or sheep, and *wal* meaning "one who takes care of".

☆ The name "Bakarwal" implies "high-altitude goatherds/shepherds".

☆ They are migratory animals and usually dark coloured, spotted coat, with strong body.

☆ Horned animals, resistant to nutritional stress as well as diseases.

☆ Usually breed twice a year and twins are not uncommon.

☆ Buck weighs from 55-65 kgs and doe from 45-50 kg.

BARBARI

☆ This is short haired and erect-horned goat popular in urban areas of Delhi, Uttar Pradesh, Gurgaon, Karnal, Panipat and Rohtak in Haryana state.

☆ Barbari breeds are grown mainly for milk and meat purpose.

☆ The color of this breed is white with light brown patches.

☆ An adult female goat weighs between 25kgs to 35kgs, whereas an adult male goat ranges between 35kgs to 45kgs.

☆ They are having the ability to give 1 kg to 1.5kgs of milk per day.

☆ This breed have better reproductive capabilities and will give, 2 to 3 kids in parturition.

☆ They are prolific breeder and kid twice in 12-15 months.

BEETAL

☆ It is found mainly in the state of Punjab

☆ These breeds are grown mainly for the purpose of milk and meat.

☆ Generally smaller than the breed of Jamunapari.

☆ Coat Colour is predominantly black or brown with white spots.

☆ Males usually possess beard.

☆ Average birth weight - 3 kg.

☆ An adult female goat ranges between 40kgs to 50kgs, whereas an adult male ranges between 50kgs to 70kgs.

☆ Age at first kidding - 20-22 months.

☆ They are having the ability to give 1 kg to 2kgs of milk per day.

BLACK BENGAL

☆ The coat colour is predominantly black, brown/grey and white with soft, glossy and short hairs.

☆ Small in body size, legs are short, back is straight and both sexes are bearded.

☆ Average live weight of buck is 15 kg and doe is 12 kg.

☆ Most prolific among the Indian breeds. Multiple births are common, twins, triplets or quadruplets.

☆ Kidding is twice a year. Average litter size is 2.1.

☆ Average age at first kidding is 9-10 months.

☆ Its skin is in great demand for high quality shoe-making.

CHEGU

☆ The coat colour is predominantly white but greyish red and mixed colours are also seen.

☆ Average live weight of buck is 39 kg and doe is 26 kg.

☆ Average birth weight is 2.0 kg with kidding once a year and mostly single.

☆ Average lactation yield is 69 kg and lactation length is 187 days.

☆ Used for draught to carry salt and small loads.

☆ Legs are medium sized. Face and muzzle is tapering. Ears are small.

☆ Horns are bent upward, backward and outward with one or more twists.

CHANGTHANGI/PASHMINA GOAT

☆ It is inhabitant of cold dry arid region of Ladakh in J&K State.

☆ Predominantly white and the rest are brown, grey and black.

☆ Undercoat white/grey; yields warm delicate fibre - pashmina (cashmere).

☆ Body and legs are small, have strong body and powerful legs.

☆ Ears are small, pricked and pointed outwards.

☆ Horns are large turning outward, upward and inward forming a semicircular ring.

☆ Average live weight of buck is 20 kg and doe is 20 kg; average birth weight is 2.1 kg.

☆ Kidding is once a year, normally single.

☆ Average age at first kidding is 20 months.

JAMUNAPARI

☆ Jamunapari breeds are found mainly in the state of Uttar Pradesh.

☆ Its coat colour is white with tan or black markings at neck and ears

☆ They are bearded in both sexes; have tuft of long hairs in the buttocks.

☆ It is largest and most elegant of the long-legged goats of India.

☆ It has pronounced Roman nose having a tuft of hair which results in parrot mouth appearance.

☆ Their horns are short and flat and horizontally twisting backward.

☆ It has large folded pendulous ears which are drooped downwards.

☆ An adult female weighs between 45kgs to 60kgs, whereas an adult male ranges between 65kgs to 80kgs.

☆ Average birth weight is up to 4 kg.

☆ Average age at first kidding is 20-25 months.

☆ They have large udder and big teats and average yield of milk is 2 to 2.5kgs of milk per day.

☆ They thrive best under range conditions with plenty of shrubs for browsing.

OSMANABADI

☆ The coat colour is predominantly black; white, brown and spotted.

☆ Long and short-haired type, based on presence or absence of long hair on the thighs and hind quarters.

☆ Tall and large size body and legs.

☆ Average birth weight 2.4 kg with kidding once a year.

☆ Average age at first kidding 19-20 months.

☆ It has good quality meat.

☆ Good yielders produce up to 3.5 kg milk a day.

SIROHI

☆ The coat colour is brown, white, and admixture of colours in typical patches; hair coarse and short.

☆ Compact and medium sized body.

☆ Tail twisted and carries coarse pointed hair.

☆ Horns are small and pointed, curved upward and backward.

☆ Average body weight of buck is 50 and doe is 23 kg.Average birth weight is 2.0 kg.

☆ Kidding is once a year but twins are common.

☆ Average age at first kidding is 19 months.

☆ Average lactation yield - 71 kg with lactation length of 175 days.

TELLICHERRY/MALABARI

☆ It is found mostly in the state of Kerala.

☆ It is grown mostly for the purpose of meat.

☆ Generally seen in white, purple and black colors.

☆ An adult female ranges in weight from 30 to 40kgs, whereas an adult male ranges between 40 to 50kgs.

☆ They can yield 1 kg to 2kgs of milk per day.

☆ These types of breeds have better reproductive capabilities and can give twins or triplets.

Some of Important Exotic Goat Breeds

ALPINE

☆ Alpine can easily be found all across US. These goats were first originated in the Alps and are also commonly known as "French Alpine."

☆ These goats range for medium to large size and adapt to their environment very easily.

☆ They come in various colors and patterns.

☆ Alpines are one of the best for dairy farming as their milk contains an average of 3.5 per cent butterfat.

☆ The goats are seasonal breeders.

ANGORA

☆ Angoras are raised for their thick fleece.

☆ They are medium sized goats having long thick coat also known as mohair.

☆ They have a Turkish background.

BOER GOAT

☆ Boer goat is a breed of goat that was developed in South Africa in the early 1900s for meat production.

☆ They were selected for meat rather than milk production; due to selective breeding and improvement.

☆ Boer goat has a fast growth rate and excellent carcass qualities, making it one of the most popular breeds of meat goat in the world.

☆ Boer goats commonly have white bodies and distinctive brown heads.

☆ Does are reported to have superior mothering skills as compared to other.

☆ Boer goats tend to gain weight at about the same rate as their sire.

☆ Kids reach marketing age at weaning attaining weight from 30-36 kgs.

LAMANCHA

☆ LaMancha have a Spanish origin but are easily found in US.

☆ They are medium in size and healthy, friendly and sturdy goats.

☆ They have the best dairy temperament and thus, provide rich dairy produce.

☆ Their milk contains about 4.2 per cent of butterfat.

☆ They are also seasonal breeders.

☆ LaMancha are medium sized goats with small tiny ears that are either gopher ears (sweet rolls) or elf ears (hooked ears).

NIGERIAN DWARFS

☆ The Nigerian goats, as the name suggests, originated from Africa.

☆ They are tiny, small goats best for dairy produce. Although they are very small but can give up to 3-4 pounds of milk per day.

☆ They are regarded to be the best dairy goats as their milk contains about 6.1 per cent butterfat.

☆ These goats also come in variety of colors and patterns.

NUBIAN

☆ Nubians also known as Anglo-Nubian are big, graceful goats.

☆ They are proud of their body structure as they have long, pendulum-like ears and Roman nose.

☆ They are a cross breed of African and Indian bucks and were raised in England.

☆ Although, they are large in size but are not heavy producers.

☆ Their milk approximately contains 4.6 per cent of butterfat.

☆ They are considered seasonal breeders but they can even be raised all year round.

PASHMINA OR CHANGTHANGI

☆ It is a breed of goat inhabiting the plateaus in Tibet and neighbouring areas of Ladakh in Jammu and Kashmir.

☆ The habitat of Pashmina goats is spread throughout the mountaineers regions of Central Asia.

☆ They are raised for ultra-fine cashmere or pashmina, measuring between 12-14 microns but were also reared for meat in the past.

☆ These goats are generally domesticated and are reared by nomadic communities called the Changpa in the Changthang region of Greater Ladakh.

☆ The goats produce a double fleece consisting of the fine, soft undercoat of hair mingled with a straighter and much coarser outer coating of hair called guard hair.

☆ These goats are of medium type, their height ranges from 60 - 80 centimeters. The average weight of male and female Pashmina goats is about 45 and 35 kilograms respectively.

☆ They possess wide, long curved horns, have blocky builds, and refined features.

SAANEN

☆ They are large, white goats with upright ears and originally grown in Switzerland.

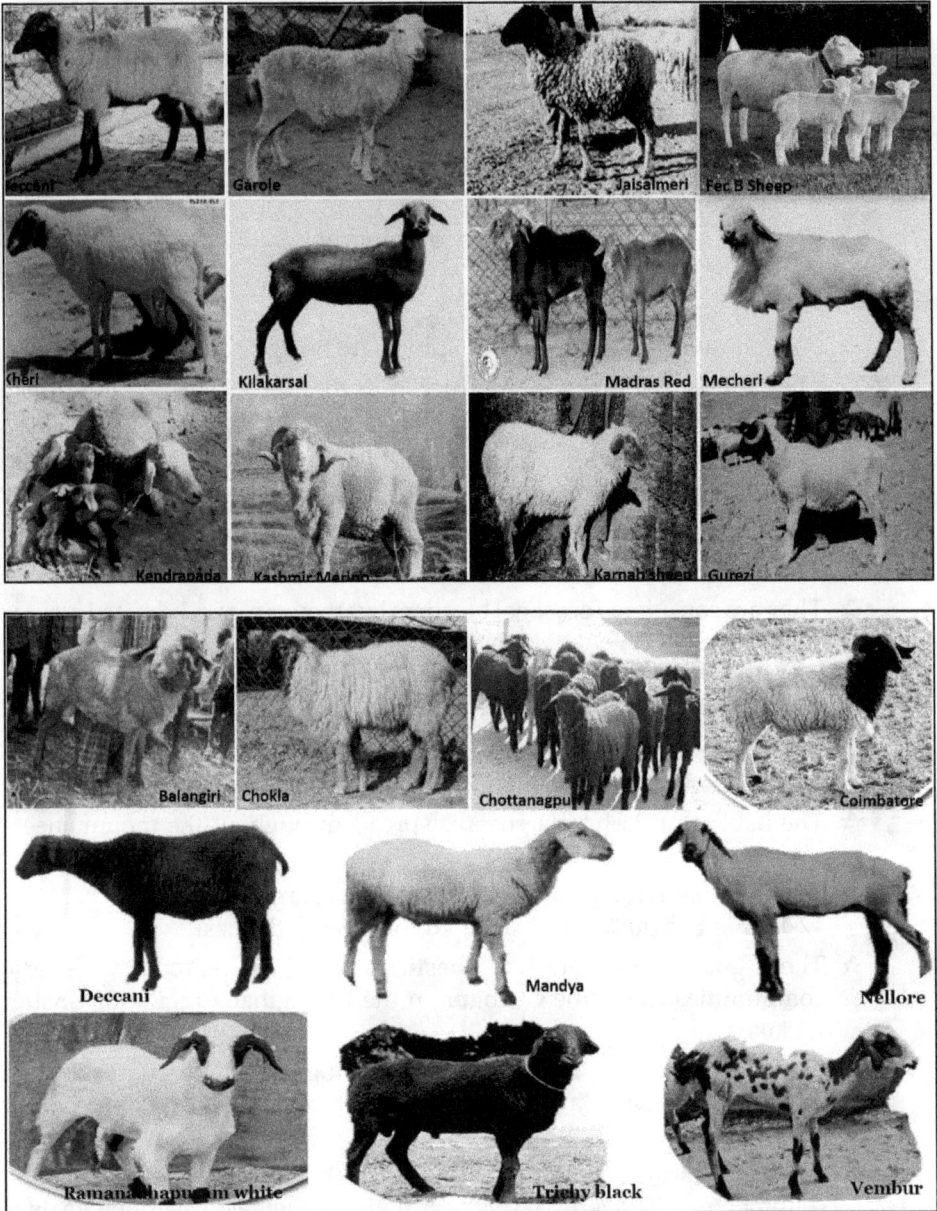

Pictures of some important Sheep Breeds.

☆ Saanen goats are heavy producers but their milk is low in butterfat as compared to other dairy goats.

SPANISH MEAT GOAT

☆ Also known as Brush goats, they were introduced in America by Europeans.

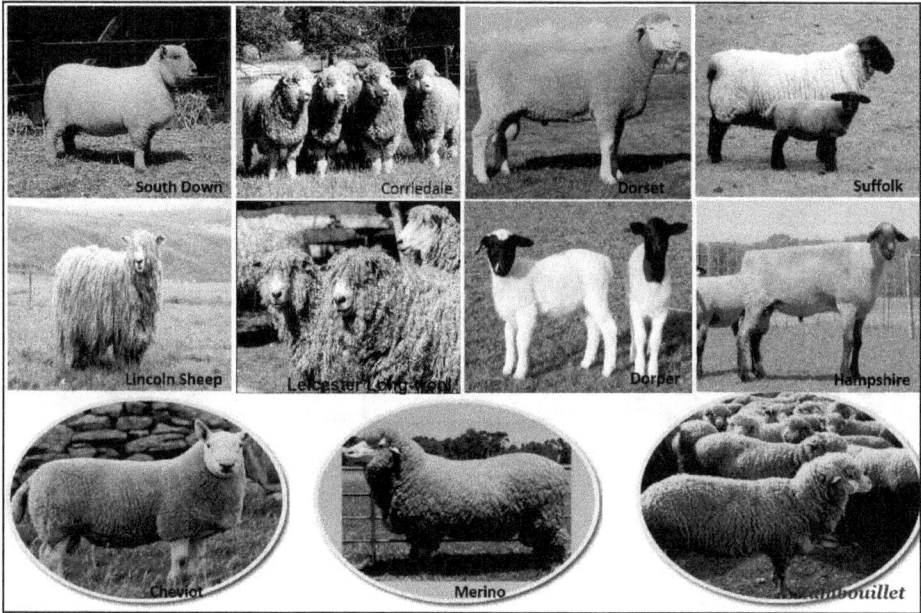

Pictures of some important Sheep Breeds.

- ✰ They are short but have a strong built.
- ✰ These meat goats are available in various colors and can be grown in any month of the year.

TENNESSEE FAINTING GOAT

- ✰ These goats have various names due to their unique characteristics.
- ✰ The most popular ones are fainting or nervous goats named after their genetic imbalance.
- ✰ When shocked or surprised, these goats fall down as their muscles get locked or jammed.
- ✰ Nevertheless, they not only provide generous amount of meat but also fleece.

TOGGENBURG GOAT

- ✰ They are the oldest breed of dairy goats having medium-sized body.
- ✰ They come in various colors ranging from fawn to dark chocolate brown with white marks on the body.
- ✰ They are commonly raised for producing milk which is usually used to make cheese. However, their milk contains only 3.3 per cent of butterfat.

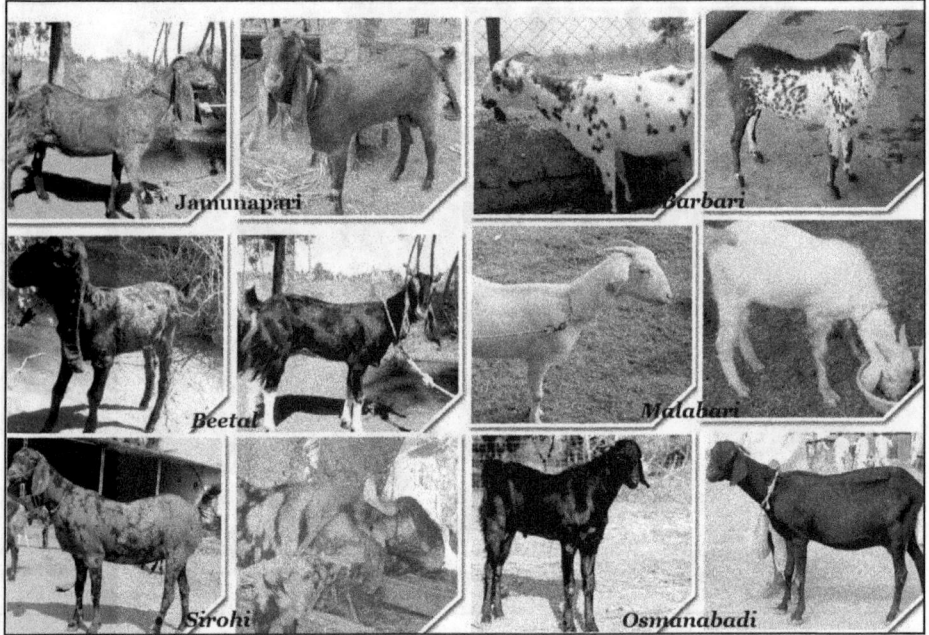

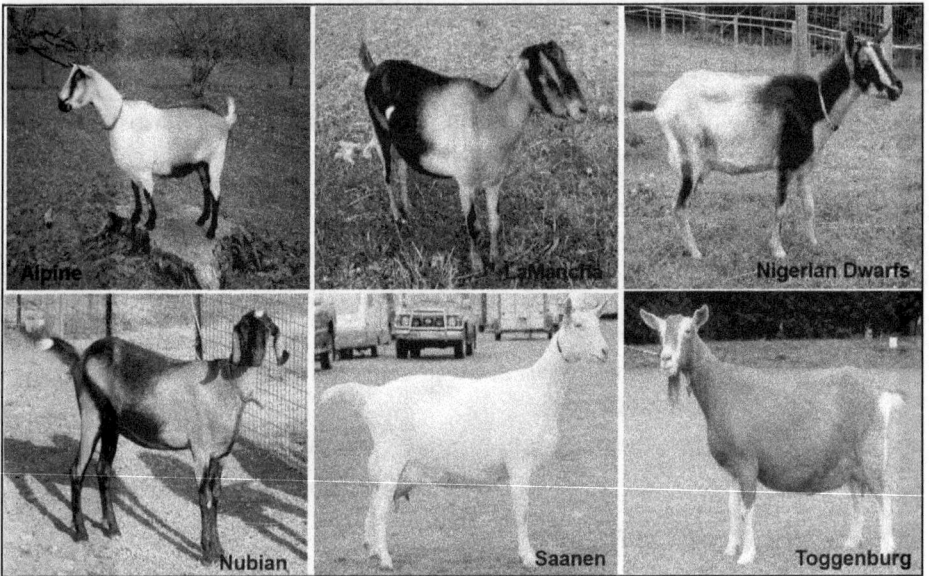

Pictures of some Important Goat Breeds.

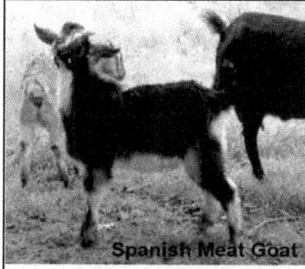
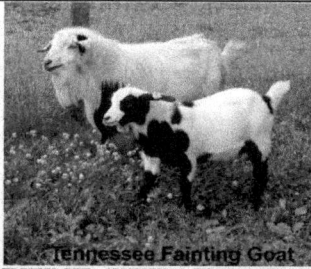
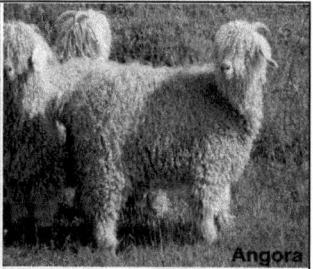
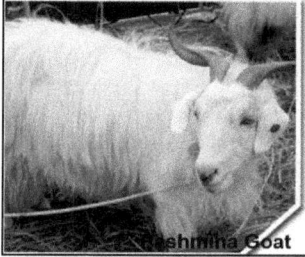
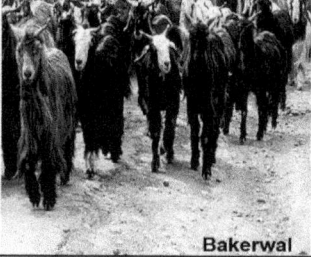
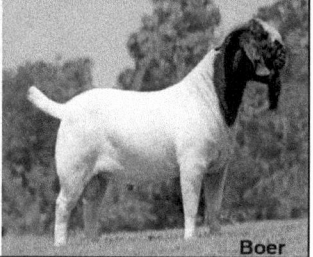

Pictures of some Important Goat Breeds.

Chapter 8

Management of Farm Records

Keeping farm records are essential for efficient and effective functioning of the farm. A producer may well know a lot about the animals he keeps. However, keeping the information in ones memory is not reliable enough; anybody can easily forget something, therefore, keeping written records helps to avoid loss of useful information. Record keeping is an essential part of good animal farm business management. From the records pedigree is ascertained and implementation of breeding programme for improvement of the herd becomes easy. Farm records help in keeping track of various farm activities viz vaccinations, medications, feeding and other farm efficiency indicators. Record keeping enables farmer to plan for economical feeding of animals, culling of under-productive animals, stocking and sale of products, and finally computation of financial data. Records should be stored in a place where it will not become soiled or damaged thus making the records useless. The format should be simple and readily understood.

Types of Records

There are numerous types of records that can be kept at a farm. However, the producer should keep record of relevant information limited to that can be utilized. There are two general categories of sheep/goat farm records.

1. **Production records**: Production records for a sheep and goat enterprise should, for example, consist of information on herd health, performance of the herd as well as the performance of the individuals within the herd over successive years. These records should also include information on fertility, prolificacy, rearing or mothering ability and production traits like milk, lamb/kid growth rate.

2. **Financial records**: Primarily relate to money or economic interactions on the farm. There are some institutions that will require detailed business and personal information on all farm assets as well as the status of

unpaid financial obligations. Financial records justify or prove farm income or expense transactions. Examples of financial records are product sales,operating expenses (feed cost, veterinary expenses, forage seeds *etc.*), equipment purchases,accounts payable, inventories, depreciation records, loan balances and price information.

General Principles of Record Keeping

☆ All records, must be accurate, neat and complete, which is achieved by filling them in as soon as possible after the operation or transaction and by checking them regularly. If possible records should be kept every day.

☆ Accurate measurement of quantities. It is of no use to guess the quantities, things should be measured and weighed properly by standard instruments.

☆ Use the records for improvement, there is absolutely no value in spending time on records and calculations of profit and production if not used. All the results should be compared with some standards, and it could be the results for previous years or the results for other farms, to improve the management.

Animal Identification

Record keeping begins with individual animal identification. The ideal animal identification is one that is permanent, resistant to loss or tearing, easy to read, and easy to apply. Choice of identification will depend upon owner's preference, needs, cost, and retention rate in the animal. Commonly used identification tools are Tagging, Branding, Tattooing.

Tagging

Tags are mostly applied in ear of the animal and do come in many different sizes, designs and brands. There are brass, aluminum, and plastic tags; button tags, rotary tags, swivel tags, and looping tags; DNA tags, and RFID (electronic tags).

Metal tags are the cheapest and easiest to apply, but they are more likely to be ripped out and cause a reaction in the ear. Brass tags are ideal for tagging small or newborn lambs. They are light, so they will not pull down on the ear. However, the lamb must be caught in order to read its tag.

Swivel and looping tags work well for lambs and are easier to read than brass tags. Temple tags have an open end to prevent ripping of the ear. However, you must punch a hole in the ear before inserting the tag. Visual plastic tags are two-piece, that come in many different sizes, shapes, and colors. They are easier to read than other tag types. Retention is fairly good, but declines with larger tag sizes. Most companies make smaller tags for sheep and lambs. Ear tags should be placed between the middle and lower cartilage ribs in the ear and far enough out on the ear to allow for later wool growth.Different colored tags can be used for different birth years, breed types, sires, or owners. The name or registration prefix of the producer or farm can be written or imprinted on the tag. Ear tags can be inserted in different ears (right or left) to denote sex of the lamb or breed type.

Tattooing

Tattoos are the best permanent form of identification. They also do not harm the animal's appearance or reduce its value in any way. The numbers and letters are made of needles that place small holes in the ears in their shape and the ink is applied to the holes so that the number is readable. The biggest disadvantage to tattooing is that tattoos are difficult to read from a distance. It is usually necessary to catch the animal for reading tattoos.

Ear Notching

An ear notch is a V-shaped notch placed somewhere in the ear. Ear notching in sheep is more commonly used for simple differentiation. For example, to denote birth type and/or week of birth or to mark ewes for culling.

Neck Chains or Straps

Neck chains or straps are the least used form of identification in sheep. They are most common with dairy animals. Neck chains have a numbered tag that corresponds to that animal's identification number. The chain is positioned around the animals neck tight enough not to fall off, but loose enough to allow for easy breathing and growth of young animals. Chains can be caught on protrusions that may choke an animal. They are difficult to see when animals are in a group. They are not a form of permanent identification since they can be easily removed.

Electronic ID (RFID)

The number of animals being identified with radio frequency identification (RFID) technology is rapidly growing. RFID system has a microchip that is a form of identification that is implanted in an electronic chip with a miniature radio transponder and antenna, under the skin of an animal. The most common implant site is between the shoulder blades or near the base of the ear.A microchip is encapsulated in a standard plastic ear tag. A microchip can also be administered as a rumen bolus using a balling gun and resides in the reticulum of the animal. Electronic ear tags are the most common form of electronic ID. It is a sure technique to identify animal easily without any handling of animal. It also provides details of the animal that are memorized/stored in the microchip. However, it is not cost effective.

National Animal ID

A national systems for animal identification is still being developed in our country. Its purpose is to trace movements of animals, in the event of a disease outbreak or act of bioterrorism. Most other developed countries have similar systems in place.

Temporary ID

Sometimes, temporary identification is desirable in a sheep flock. Paint

Following format of different record registers could be of value in any livestock enterprise.

Ewe/Goat Record

Ewe No./Doe No.	Sire No.	Sire Breed	Dam No.	Dam Breed	Date of Birth	Birth Weight	Type of Birth (S/T/Tr)	Type of Rearing	Age and Weight at Weaning	Shorn Fleece Weight	Lamb Details	Remarks

S: Single; T: Twins; Tr: Triplets.

Ram/Buck Record

Ram/Buck No.	Sire No.	Sire Breed	Dam No.	Dam Breed	Date of Birth	Birth Weight	Type of Birth (S/T/Tr)	Type of Rearing	Age and Weight at Weaning	Shorn Fleece Weight	Progeny Performance	Remarks

S: Single; T: Twins; Tr: Triplets.

Lambing or Kidding Record

Year	Flock Cate- gory	Date Ram Tur- ned in	Date Ram Tur- ned Out	Ram ID	Ewe ID	Date of Lam- bing	Lamb ID	Sex	Type of Birth	Body Col- our	Body Cover	Birth Wt.	Wt. at 2 wks	Wt. at 1 Mon- th	Wt. at 2nd Mon- th	Wt. at Wean- ing	Date of Wean- ing	Nurs- ing Abil- ity	Date of Cast- ration	Market Wt.	Dis- posal Mode	Dis- posal Date	Rem- arks

Breeding Record

Dam ID	Dam Breed	Sire ID	Sire Breed	Dam Parity	Mating Date 1st	Mating Date 2nd	Lambing/ Kidding Date	Lambing/ Kidding Type S/T/Tr	Remarks

S: Single; T: Twins; Tr: Triplets.

Lamb/Kid Performance Record

						Pre-weaning						Weaning				
Lamb/Kid ID	Breed	Sex	Date of Birth	Type of Birth S/T/Tr	Birth Wt.	Body Measurement at birth WHt/BL/HG	Feeding Type	Weaning Date	Weaning Wt.	Type of Rearing	Body Measurements at weaning WHt/BL/HG	Age at Marketing	Wt. at Marketing	BCS (1-5)	Price at Marketing

S: Single; T: Twins; Tr: Triplets; WHt: Wither height; BL: Body length; HG: Heart girth.

Animal Health Record

Animal ID	Breed	Sex	Date of Observation	Major Signs	Suspected Disease	Treatment given	Duration of Medication	Response	Remarks

Vaccination Record

Animal ID	Breed	Name/Type of Vaccine	Date of Vaccination	Date of Booster/Next	Remarks

Mortality Record

Animal ID	Breed	Sex	Age	Date of death	Previous Treatment if any	Remarks

Wool Production Register

Date	Wool Growth (Days)	Sides		Shoulder		Belly		Thigh		Total Yield	Grease Weight	Per cent of Yield	Clean Weight
		Fineness	Yield	Fineness	Yield	Fineness	Yield	Fineness	Yield				

Disposal Record

ID No.	Flock Category	Date of Birth/ Purchase	Single/ Twin	Sire No.	Dam No.	Date of Disposal	Wt. at Disposal	Age at Disposal	Reasons of Disposal	Remarks

branding; marking crayons, sticks, and spray markers can all be used to identify sheep and lambs for periods of several weeks to several months. Marks from marking crayons will usually last for several weeks, whereas paint brands tend to last for many months. Numbers are paint branded or spray painted on an animal's back or side for easy identification. The same number can be put on the lambs' backs so that ewe-lamb pairs can easily be identified. Paint brands allow for quick identification. Paint branding is useful for sales and exhibition because it is temporary identification that is easily visible and easy to identify animals in a sale. When paint branding wool-producing sheep, only wool colours are applied. Heavy applications should be avoided because excess paint makes it difficult to scour the wool.

Chapter 9

Fodder Management

Livestock sector is dependent on feed, fodder and forage availability. The livestock rearing has remained and still remains confined to rural areas for the reason that fodder is available in these areas. A great chunk of land in rural areas has been dedicated to the livestock grazing only, termed as "Gass Charai" and part of cultivable land is used for fodder crops. Interestingly many staple/oil crops have been replaced by fodder crops due to high demand of fodder. The scarcity of fodder was not much concern earlier but it is now an important issue in livestock farming. The land availability per capita has drastically reduced, cultivable land is squeezing day by day due to urbanization, Gass charai land is no more available in the villages that has been mostly grabbed by land mafia. The tremendous growth in livestock sector due to enormous surge in population growth and increasing demands for foods of animal origin has put pressure on fodder availability. India today is 40 per cent deficit in dry fodder, 36 per cent in green fodder and 57 per cent in concentrates which warrants technologies that can on one hand conserve the surplus fodder during flush periods (spring and monsoon) and on the other hand increase the quality of fodders for animal consumption during lean periods of hot summer or winter.

The major important Kharif forage crops are;

    i. Fodder Maize – (African Tall)

    ii. Sorghum - (MP Chari)

    iii. Cowpea – (Bundel lobia 1or UPC-9202)

Major important Rabi crops are;

    i. Oats – (Sabzar)

    ii. Berseem – (BL-180)

    iii. Winter Vetch – (Golden Tares)

Important perennial forage crops are;

    i. Orchard Grass – (currie)

    ii. Tall Fescue – (Demeter)

    iii. Rye Grass – (Manawa)

    iv. Clover – Red/White (Montogomery/Ladino)

    v. Sainfoin – (Melrose)

    vi. Lucerne – (S-9)

Ruminants in general are fed poor quality roughages with little nutritive value, however, in tropical environments sheep and goats have to eat feeds that contain a lot of fiber during most parts of the year. The bulky and fibrous nature of coarse feeds results in poor nutrient supply and reduced intake. Such feeds have to remain in the rumen for extended periods of time before they are sufficiently digested to move out of the rumen and allow more feed consumption. It is common for animals to lose weight and condition, produce less and even have difficulty breeding when fed on these low quality roughages.

Several technologies have been developed to enhance the nutritive value of poor quality forages which include physical treatment (ball milling, steaming, chopping), chemical treatment (urea or ammonia treatment, alkali treatment) or enzymatic treatment or fungal treatment. Treatment of roughages, either physically or chemically, is aimed at rendering the structural constituents more accessible to microbial digestive enzymes in the rumen.

Physical Treatment

The main objective of this method is to reduce the size of the roughage to expose more surface area for microbial degradation in the rumen. This involves hydration (soaking) and chopping.

Soaking Coarse Crop Residues such as Maize Stover

Dryness increases time spent chewing per bolus and thus reduces total intake. However, hydration has a potential to overcome these constraints. Soaking causes swelling of cell-wall structures, making them more accessible to cellulolytic microbes. In addition, it reduces the dustiness and dryness of the feed. Soaking per se has potential to overcome some of the constraints to intake of maize stover. The voluntary feed intake of chopped maize stover can be improved by 23 per cent by just increasing moisture content from 30 to 60 per cent. Supplementation with 5 per cent linseed meal (fermentable nitrogen source) doubled the consumption of the stovers.

Chopping

    ☆ Chopped fodder can be easily eaten.

    ☆ Chopping also minimizes selection and facilitates mixing with other feeds.

    ☆ Chopping can be done using a machete knife or by special manual or motor-driven choppers that are very efficient.

⭐ Moistening chopped dry roughages can also improve utilization through increasing intake and digestibility.

⭐ Chopping being an easy practice has been largely adopted by the farmers, small as well as commercial farmers.

Chemical Methods

They are relatively efficient and easy to put into practice. The effects of chemical treatment include hydrolysis of chemical bonds that involve lignin. The chemicals used in treatment of roughages are mainly alkalis. The most effective alkali is sodium hydroxide or caustic soda. It is, however, not commonly used due to its high cost and risk of use. The most common methods of chemical treatment use either ammonia or urea, which are relatively less effective but are cheaper and less hazardous to use. Moreover, treatment with ammonia or urea has the added advantage of improving the nitrogen content of the treated roughage. Treatment is recommended where roughage constitutes over half the diet or where higher levels of production are desired. The type of treatment will depend on local circumstances. Ammonia treatment is suitable for large operations such as cooperatives in areas where there is a supply of anhydrous ammonia and where the necessary infrastructure of tankers is available for its distribution. The application of this treatment method has low applicability. Urea treatment is more applicable for smaller quantities of roughage treated on small farms. Urea treatment of crop residues is being practiced.

Ammonia Treatment

⭐ Ammonia (anhydrous, gaseous) treatment requires a supply of industrially produced ammonia together with a distribution network.

⭐ Amount of ammonia used is 2.5–3.5 kg per 100 kg DM of straw.

⭐ Generally, a longer period of treatment is required at low temperatures and shorter period at higher temperatures.

⭐ Optimum moisture level for successful treatment is between 15 and 25 per cent.

⭐ An air tight seal is required.

⭐ Low-digestible roughages are treated.

Urea Treatment

⭐ Since fertilizer-grade urea is readily available, thus urea treatment is a preferred treatment technique for improving the nutritional quality of low-quality roughages (LQR) such as crop residues and agro-industrial by products.

⭐ The simplicity of its application is an added advantage of this technique.

⭐ Ammonia is released through urea degradation caused by the action of micro-organisms, which are normal inhabitants of low quality roughages that produce urease in the presence of moisture. With adequate moisture and suitable temperature, urea is degraded to ammonia which then permeates through the straw. Nitrogen released through this process is bound to the straw, thus increasing the total nitrogen content.

☆ Digestibility of the fibrous low quality roughage is also increased by the action of the treatment.

☆ Urea treatment improves the crude protein content (from 5 per cent to 10 per cent), digestibility (from 45 per cent to 50 per cent) and intake of low quality roughages by 20-40 per cent.

☆ The most common recommended level of urea is 5 kg per 100 kg of material (5 per cent urea measured on air-dry LQR). The moisture or water level in the LQR to be treated determines how much water should be added.

☆ Water is added to achieve a final moisture content of 30 per cent. It may range from 0.3 to 1 litre of water per kg straw with the minimum being applied in areas with water scarcity.

☆ An appropriate level of water is necessary for effective urea treatment as well as packing of the material to exclude air. However, care should be taken to avoid use of excess water as it will lead to risk of mold growth and leaching of urea to the bottom of the pit or trench.

☆ With some experience, the initial dry matter content of LQR can be estimated by handling. A very dry material (*i.e.*, 90 or 95 per cent dry matter) is brittle and does not stick to the hands. Conversely, a wetter residue (*i.e.*, 85 per cent dry matter) feels a little sticky and moist. It also tends to bend rather than break easily.

☆ Approximately 30 litres of water are added to LQR with 90 per cent DM and only 23 litres with 85 per cent DM to achieve 30 per cent moisture.

☆ Urea is added to the required quantity of water and mixed that is then sprinkled on the LQR as it is added to the pit in different batches. A good way of doing this is to add 10 kg of residue and then sprinkle the appropriate amount of urea-water solution.

☆ After each batch of LQR and urea-water solution is added to the pit, there should be thorough mixing with a stirring rod/stick or by hand so that the solution is uniformly spread on to the LQR to be treated. This can be done in the pit or on a plastic sheet on the ground prior to packing in the pit.

☆ A 1 × 2 × 1 m pit will typically hold between 150 and 200 kg of common LQR, with the top of the pile being at or slightly above ground level.

☆ The pit should not allow air or rain water to enter the LQR being treated. Therefore, the pit is typically lined with material such as heavy plastic.

☆ An airtight condition is easily achieved by applying a plastic cover. When straw is stacked against firm structures (walls, inside pits, meshed wire), it can be compacted by trampling. Wet straw compacts better and will not allow air to enter. Chopping LQR such as maize and sorghum stover before treatment helps better compaction and treatment.

☆ A concrete pit, placed above ground, lined with plastic will produce a good result, but may be too expensive, in which case, other alternatives are used.

☆ Apart from pits or trenches, plastic bags can be used that can hold 20–25 kg of treated straw. Such bags have an advantage in that individual bags can be opened when they are actually needed to feed animals.

☆ A number of factors influence the length of time needed for most effective urea treatment. One of the most important is outside temperature. Higher temperatures lessen the length of time needed, and cooler temperatures increase the length of time required. It is commonly recommended that the pit remain closed for at least 3 weeks, and preferably 1 month.

☆ Well-treated roughages will have a uniform, dark-brown colour throughout the treated material and a strong pungent smell of ammonia.

The other approach in fodder management is preserving surplus fodder received during lush periods of the year for its use in livestock during lean periods. Two important technologies involved are;

   i. Hay making

   ii. Silage making

Hay Making

The most commonly practiced method for conservation of fodder is hay making. It is simple wherein green fodder is subjected to sun drying till its moisture content is reduced to not more than 15 per cent. However, the success of traditional hay making depends upon the chance selection of a period of fine weather. More recently introduction of rapid drying techniques using barn drying equipments have significantly improved the efficiency of the process and reduced the dependence on weather. In such case forage is allowed to meet hot gasses at temperatures of about 150 °C for 20 to 50 minutes depending upon drier design and moisture content of crop. Though the water content in the forage reduces as it matures, but more matured green forages are low in nutritive value so matured forages are not suitable for hay making. Good quality hay provides a considerable proportion of energy and certain other essential nutrients like carotene. Natural, local, improved grasses or legumes like oats, orchard grass, Lucerne, berseem, tall fesue cowpea and even clovers are all suitable for hay making. Thick stemmed forages require chopping before drying. For hay making the leguminous crops must be cut in pre-blossom stage in order to conserve protein and available energy. Chemical changes arising from action of plant and microbial enzymes, chemical oxidation, leaching and mechanical damage results in inevitable losses of valuable nutrients during the drying process. The magnitude of these losses depend largely on speed of drying. A number of devices and methods are used to speed up the drying process in the field which include çonditioners" such as crushers, rollers and crimpers which break the cellular structures of the plant and allow the air to penetrate swath more easily. In hay making the biggest loss is in terms of loss of leaves particularly in case of legumes like berseem, Lucerne. To minimize the loss some measures must be observed like:

    i. Cut the crop in pre-blossom stage

    ii. Chop the forage while still moist. Chopping should not be fine, 5-8 cm length is recommended.

    iii. Spread wet chopped forage in sun on smooth hard surface in thin layer.

    iv. Turn the forage every 2-3 hours during the day. Under exposure to sun.

    v. Within 2-3 days forage will be dry depending upon turning as well as exposure to sun and air movement.

    vi. Gather the dried stems and leaves to store or marketing. If bailers are available chopped dried fodder can be bailed for easy transport and shall reduce store space.

    vii. Hay is rich in nutrients and 130 kg hay containing 90 per cent dry matter shall be equal to 600 kg green forage containing 15 per cent dry matter.

The losses associated with hay making do not completely cease when hay is stored. The stored crop may contain 10 to 30 per cent moisture. At higher moisture levels, chemical changes brought about by enzymes and microorganisms are likely to occur. The chemical oxidation in the hay releases heat when stocked that may sometimes make hay vulnerable to combustion. Prolonged heating during storage may have adverse effect on proteins of hay, new linkages are formed which may prove resistant to hydrolysis by proteases, therefore reducing solubility and digestibility of proteins in hay. Carotene losses are observed during storage of hay and in general proportion of cell wall constituents are increased and nutritive value decreases with storage of hay. These losses in the hay during storage can be reduced through application of hay preservatives. The preservatives include propionic acid applied at the rate of 10g/kg water or 3kg/ton of forage with 30 per cent moisture content. It should be applied in sufficient quantity and distributed uniformly. Lactic acid producing bacteria have also been used with less effect. More recently anhydrous ammonia application in plastic covered stacks or bales of moist hay has increased stability and improved nutritive value of hay but has a risk of toxicity so cautiously employed.

Silage Preparation

It is an important method of conserving green fodder for livestock in situations like drought, heavy rainfall or scarcity of fodder. It is preservation of chaffed cereal green fodder in anaerobic condition by way of controlled fermentation. The anaerobic condition is achieved by chopping the crop during harvesting, then rapid filling of silo pits or tanks and by adequate consolidation and sealing. Sealing is must to prevent re-entry and circulation of air during storage. In anaerobic condition the sugars contained in green fodder are converted to lactic acid by microorganisms that preserve the fodder for long periods. Here the green fodder which is put in silage pits or tanks in air tight condition, oxygen is utilized by living cells in chaffed green fodder and carbon dioxide and water is released, carbon dioxide pushes air out and also restricts growth of organism dependent of oxygen as well as undesirable microbes like clostridia and enterobacteria, thus preserves fodder for long periods some 6 months to a year.

For silage making the suitable fodder crops are green fodder maize, sorghum, bajra, oats, orchard grass, tall fescue *etc.* which are rich in soluble carbohydrates. Preference is given to cereal green fodders (monocotyledons) because they contain more sugar content which is utilized in fermentation process to make lactic acid by microorganisms. These types of crops have hard and big stems and are not suitable for hay making but best suited for silage preparation. The attainment of critical pH for silage preparation is more difficult with crops of high buffering capacity like legumes. Silage making has some plus points over hay making like;

i. Silage requires less space for storage as it is pressed in pit/tank.

ii. Silage is prepared in closed, air tight condition so no danger of fire.

iii. Thick stemmed forages which are difficult to conserve as hay can be conserved more conveniently and efficiently as silage.

iv. Ensilaging is less dependent on weather fluctuations.

v. The digestibility of forage is improved due to partial breakdown of structural carbohydrates, and presence of lactic acid reserves the energy of animals for production as lactic acid is easily digestible to animals.

vi. Silage is tasty and flavoured so increases appetite of animals.

vii. Field losses that are experienced in hay making are reduced in silage preparation.

viii. Silage making is less labour and time consuming practice of fodder preservation.

The type of silo in which silage is prepared are very varied and range from small plastic bags to large cylindrical towers built of concrete, steel or wood.

There are two methods of silage preparation; pit method and tank method.

Before you plan for silage making, it is necessary to work out your needs. One cubic foot tank or pit will have 16 kg of chaffed green fodder in it and depending upon your requirement, accordingly pit or tank is made.

For pit method, select location at higher level on ground so that rain water does not percolate into the pit. In rectangular pit, corner edges should be made round. So that while filling and pressing fodder, air will not remain inside the pit or tank. Walls of the pit or tank should be air proof that can be achieved by plastering of silo pits with cement. If water table is high, then it is better to have silage tank than pit. Pit or tank can also be wrapped with plastic paper (200 microns) in inside out position.

When fodder is in cob stage or tussling stage, harvest it for silage making. Too mature stage is not recommended as it reduces sugar content and increases fibre content in the fodder. After harvesting the fodder let it dry for 5-6 hours in shed so that its moisture content decreases from 80 per cent to 65-70 per cent. Avoid silage making during rainy days. Following few points should be observed while silage making.

 i. Prior to filling silage pit or tank, clean and dry it.

 ii. Cover with plastic film inside in such a way that it covers all four sides of the pit/tank.

 iii. Chaff the fodder to 2 cm length for filling silo pit.

 iv. Prepare separate solution of urea, jaggary, mineral mixture and common salt in 15-20 liters and spread it on layer of pressed chaffed green fodder.

 v. After making 4th thick layer of chaffed green fodder, press it with wooden planks or motars in such a way that air will not entangle in chaffed fodder. Then sprinkle solution of urea, jaggary and mineral mixture.

 vi. Follow the same procedure until filling of pit/tank 1-1.5 feet above the ground level. Then cover it with plastic film from all sides.

 vii. Cover it with trash, straw, soil and dry hay to protect it from entering rain water into it. You may have temporary roofing of the pits to avoid rain water.

 viii. After 45- 60 days good quality silage will be ready for feeding of animals.

 ix. Good quality silage has sweet and sour taste and fruity smell. It has faint green to brownish colour and pH of 3.5 to 4.2.

 x. Poor or rotten silage has mold growth and black colour.

In ensilaging there are nutrient losses that may vary with the duration of cutting of crops and ensilaging. When the crops are ensiled on the same day of cut, nutrient losses are negligible and even over a 24 hours wilting period, losses of dry matter may occur to the tune of 1-2 per cent. However, dry matter losses may go as high as 6 per cent after 5 days of wilting or 10 per cent after 8 days of wilting in the field and water soluble carbohydrates and proteins are main nutrients affected. Effluent losses are reported in most silos and the amount of effluent produced depend largely upon initial moisture content of the crop, however, dry matter, type of silo, degree of consolidation and nature of the crop will all affect the effluent loss. Ensiling crops with dry matter content of about 15 per cent may result into effluent dry matter losses as high as 10 per cent whereas crops wilted to 30 per cent dry matter may have no effluent loss.

Silages may be classified into;

 1. Naturally fermented

  a. Unwilted well preserved silages

  b. Wilted well preserved silages and

  c. Badly preserved silages

 2. Additive treated

  a. Fermentation stimulant additives

  b. Fermentation inhibitor additives

Well preserved unwilted silages are commonly made from grasses and whole cereal crops and lactic acid bacteria dominate the fermentation. They are characterized by having low pH between 3.7 to 4.2, contain high concentrations of lactic acid, small amounts of acetic acid, traces of propionic and butyric acid and variable amounts of ethanol and mannitol. Nitrogenous compounds are in the form of soluble non-protein compounds in contrast to proteins in fresh forage crops. Gross energy of these silages is higher than those of parent material resulting from the formation of high energy compounds like ethanol.

In wilted silages, the crop prior to ensilaging is wilted that increases dry matter content and restricts the growth of undesirable microbes like closdridia and enterobacteria. The wilting restricts the fermentation as dry matter increases thus the silage is having higher pH and lower levels of fermentation acids as compared to unwilted silage and the gross energy contents are normally similar to those of parent material.

Badly preserved silages refer to the silages in which either closdridia or enterobacteria or both have dominated the fermentation. These silages are being offered to the animals but the silages deteriorated by aerobic oxidation are liable to be toxic thus not offered to the animals. Badly preserved silages are frequently produced from crops that are either ensiled at too high moisture content or contained low levels of water soluble carbohydrates. They are also produced if the ensiled forage is deficient in lactic acid bacteria. Such silages usually have high pH within the range of 5- 7, with main fermentation acids as acetic or butyric acids whereas lactic acid concentrations are low. Ammonia and degradation products such as amines and keto acids are also present in badly preserved silages.

In additive treated silages, sugar rich materials, inoculants and enzymes that encourage development of lactic acid bacteria are used as stimulants of fermentation. Molasses is one of the earliest silage fermentative stimulant that increases dry matter and lactic acid contents, and reduce pH and ammonia levels in the silage. A number of commercial inoculants containing freeze dried cultures of homofermentative lactic acid bacteria are available and have proved effective in improving silage fermentation. The inoculation of these cultures should be atleast $10^5 - 10^6$cfu/g fresh crop. The rapid domination of the fermentation by homolactic bacteria ensures most efficient use of water soluble carbohydrates and increases chances of production of well-preserved silage. Some commercial silage additives contain enzymes mostly cellulases and hemicellulases along with an inoculum of suitable strains of lactic acid bacteria. A large number of chemical compounds have been tested as potential inhibitors of fermentation, but few are accepted for commercial use. Earlier mixtures of mineral acids usually hydrochloric and sulfuric acids were added to the crops during ensilaging in sufficient quantity to lower pH value below 4. If the process is carried out effectively, it is very efficient method of conserving nutrients. However, recently formic acid has largely replaced mineral acids. It is commonly applied in the form of an aqueous solution of ammonium tetraformate at the rate of 2.5 to 5 litres per ton of fresh crop. Formalin has also been used as a fermentation inhibitor. It is applied either alone or in combination with sulphuric or formic acid. Formalin protects the plant proteins from hydrolysis by plant enzymes or microbes in silo.

Nutritive Value of some Important Hays

Fodder	CF (g/kg)	CP (g/kg)	DCP (g/kg)	ME (MJ/kg)
Meadow grass	298	113	67	8.8
Mixed grass	301	114	63	8.6
Fescue	315	90	48	8.6
Ryegrass	305	96	48	8.9
Clover	319	143	89	8.6
Lucerne	322	165	118	8.3
Soya bean	366	156	101	7.8
Oats	329	80	41	8.5
Wheat	268	82	44	7.8

Composition and Nutritive Value of Various Types of Silages

Parameters	Unwilted Silage	Wilted Silage	Badly Preserved Silage (Lucerne)	Inoculated Silage (Lactic Acid Bacteria)	Formic Acid Treated
DM (g/kg)	186	316	131	181	184
pH	3.9	4.2	7.0	4.1	3.7
Total N (g/kg DM)	23	22.8	46	32	23
Protein N (g/kg TN)	235	289	260	407	490
Ammonia N (g/kg TN)	78	79	292	88	49
Acetic acid (g/kgDM)	36	24	114	30	15
Butyric acid (g/kgDM)	1.4	0.6	8	5	0.03
Lactic acid (g/kgDM)	102	59	13	84	44
Ethanol (g/kg DM)	12	6.4	–	7	9

Chapter 10

Manure Management

Manure is organic matter, mostly derived from animal feces. Farm animals consume forages and concentrates to produce meat and milk and manure is an inevitable by-product of this process. Common forms of animal manure include farmyard manure (FYM) or farm slurry (liquid manure). FYM also contains plant material (often straw), which has been used as bedding for animals and has absorbed the feces and urine. Liquid manure, known as slurry, is produced by more intensive livestock rearing systems where floors are concrete and no straw bedding is used. Manure contains the undigested fraction of organic matter in the diet, and generally contain > 70 per cent of dietary N, and > 65 per cent of dietary P.

Manure from different animals has different qualities for instance, sheep manure is high in nitrogen and potassium, while pig manure is relatively low in both. Both sheep and goat manures are rich in nutrients, relatively dry and in pellet form, has minimal odour, normally does not attract flies and easily handled. Manure and bedding from one goat can average around 10 pounds a day. Manure from sheep and goat fed on concentrates and hay is rich in nutrients than the one from animals fed on pastures. Manure from sheep and goats that are allowed to forage should be composted in order to avoid problems with weed seeds.

Manure is an important valuable source of organic matter for agricultural soils and may provide a major contribution to biological, physical and chemical soil quality. In addition, it is an important source of plant nutrients. The organic material in manure provides structure that makes soil easier to cultivate, less compactable, less susceptible to erosion and more likely to retain water. Manure provides nutrients that are not supplied by chemical fertilizers and also favours the microorganisms in the soil that make it more fertile and healthy. The nutrients in manure readily leach into the air, soil, and water. The value of manure can be encashed by its land application or through off-farm utilization by soil producers, crop or organic farmers, gardeners, or others.

Livestock manure had played an important role in soil fertility and crop production in traditional agriculture, however, with the, ample availability of chemical fertilizers at low costs since the 1960s, has decreased the interest in utilization of livestock manures as a source of nutrients for crops. Moreover, storage, handling, easy application, low cost, and the availability of nutrients, in particular of N, which is often more reliable, has enhanced the application of chemical fertilizers to soil instead of manure. As a consequence, animal manures are being wasted causing pollution of atmosphere and water. However, use of chemical fertilizers have raised some environmental and consumer concerns and consumers are now ready to pay more for organic agricultural produce. This trend has once again made producers to rethink of use of animal manures as a source of fertilizer in their fields and has necessitated processing of livestock manure in a way to facilitate its use on-farm or off-farm without any health and environmental hazards. Since unmanaged manure contributes nutrients, disease-causing micro-organisms, and oxygen-demanding organics to the waters, thus rendering it unsafe for consumption, recreation, agriculture, manufacturing besides disturbs the aquatic ecosystem, therefore manure management constitutes an important integral part of livestock farm management.

Manure management is as old as human history and as new as the latest adaptation of a time-honoured practice. Proper manure management benefits the producer as well as the rest of the ecosystem. Manure solids are being composted, often with urban residues such as leaves and grass clippings, to produce soil amendments high in organic-matter content. Liquid manure can be covered and anaerobically digested to capture biogas-principally methane for energy production. Keeping the manure dry reduces the opportunity for anaerobic digestion but increases the opportunity for the manure to be used as an animal feed supplement, as is being done with poultry litter as a supplement to cattle feed or in fish meals. Application of manures to the land at the proper time-using proper management techniques and in proper amounts-recycles the nutrients through the soil, reducing the expense of commercial (inorganic) fertilizers as well as the need to add organic matter. Proper manure management improves water quality by preventing pollutants such as nutrients, organics, and pathogens from percolating to the surface and ground waters. Soil quality is also improved through the addition of organic materials that improve soil tilth and increase the soil's water-holding capacity. Air quality also benefits from reduced emissions of methane and ammonia compounds, as well as reduced odours.

Often manure is stockpiled by the livestock farmers without having any awareness of proper management which leads to the seeping of these piles into water ways, wells, streams or ponds. Disposal of manure into ditches, lanes, drains or other out of way places also leads to the contamination of water posing a serious threat to the human and animal health. Therefore, proper management of manure is must to yield the benefits of manure for on or off-farm use and reduce environmental pollution and offending neighbours.

Land application of manure to fertilize crops is considered the most suitable method to utilize animal manures. land is a gigantic bio-conversion system, developed during millions of years, and able to bio-degrade animal and plant wastes to become part of the soil. Land application of manure serves two objectives one the waste disposal and the other recycling of waste components. The best responding soils generally are those with a low natural fertility. Such soils may be improved significantly by regular additions of animal manure.

Manure management encompasses various activities including pasture and paddock management, manure collection, transport, storage, handling, treatment, disposal and utilization of manure. A livestock farm should have a basic manure management plan that includes the quantity of manure and bedding generated annually on the farm, handling and collection methods, size and location of storage, composting facilities, ways and means to prevent soiling of water sources, pastures, storage areas or even paddocks. Following are few important points that should be considered while storing the manure.

☆ Manure should be collected regularly from paddocks and stalls preferably daily.

☆ Manure storage facilities do not need to be fancy. In most instances the storage area is temporary until the manure is land applied or hauled away for composting.

☆ If composting the manure, the storage area can be the compost area or bins.

☆ The storage area must be large enough to effectively hold all the manure and bedding generated until it can be utilized.

☆ Locate the storage area on high ground and away from drainage or run-off areas.

☆ Storage area should not be located in a floodplain or otherwise must be properly protected from inundation during floods.

☆ Storage area should be located at a place that is accessible to equipments like carts, tractors and manoeuvrability.

☆ Planning for long-term winter storage for 5 to 6 months (October to March) is necessary. Rainy weather and ground saturation in the fall and spring should also be considered.

☆ Manure piles should not be allowed to reach more than 8-10 feet as it may pose a fire threat.

☆ Locate the storage facility near the manure source. If manure is to be applied to crop land that is at a significant distance from the barn, a satellite storage area near the cropland may be appropriate ("field stacking").

☆ It is essential that the storage area is accessible during inclement weather.

☆ The storage area should be located at least 100 feet away from wells, potable water sources, wetlands, and surface water bodies (streams, ponds).

☆ Storage areas should be 200 feet away from residences.

☆ Do not store the manure in barns or paddocks that can serve as a potential source of parasite infestation to the livestock.

☆ Place the storage area downwind from barns and (most importantly) neighbours' residences.

☆ It is better to have manure storage area invisible to farm visitors or neighbours or otherwise consider concealing the area from view.

☆ Farms with few animals can store manure in plastic garbage cans with lids, wood or metal bins, or carts.

☆ Farms that are utilizing manure for land application can store manure and stall waste in the dumpsters that should cater the storage needs for a week or less. A truck bed, tractor trolley can be used for temporary storage for later removal to the manure storage area. It may be necessary if the storage area is located away from the barns.

☆ For most small farms, manure storage can be a pile contained on a pad or in a small shed. The use of a wooden or masonry "bucking wall" behind the pile will help in unloading and loading manure and will screen the pile from view. Reinforced concrete will be necessary for large structures.

☆ Using three bucking walls, the manure and leachate can be contained and handled more effectively and easily.

☆ Structures for storing larger quantities of manure should be designed with three or four sides, a wide opening, a high permanent roof and more durable construction either wooden or concrete.

☆ Floors of compacted earth or stone dust are adequate for farms with few livestock. Packed gravel, road base material, or crushed limestone base or reinforced concrete is recommended for farms with larger number of animals.

☆ Manure storage structures should be monitored during the wet season to determine the leachate draining from the pile and ensure its proper draining into the filter area.

☆ Slope the entrance ramp upward to keep surface water from entering.

☆ Make one side of the structure on ground level for dumping and removal of manure.

☆ Rough-surfaced ramp should be designed to lead into the storage area having sufficient width to allow farm equipments like carts, wheelbarrows, tractors or trolleys to maneuver in and out when unloading or loading.

☆ It is essential to cover the storage area to prevent run-off from the pile which can lead to water contamination. A covered area also protects the manure from losing the nutrients.

☆ Depending on the size of storage area, a watertight plastic tarp can be sufficient. However, large manure storage areas can have permanent roofs which is resistant to wind and rains.

☆ Install gutters to catch water flowing off the roof and channel them away from storage area. It is important to manage the seepage or runoff from the storage area that may lead to contamination of water and thus lead to livestock diseases.

☆ Stall waste is usually dry however, manure from paddock clean-up may contribute to the leachate that too when the bedding is not sufficient to absorb the liquid.

☆ Proper management of seepage includes construction of trenches or laying of pipes around the manure storage piles to capture the leachate and direct it to the filler/buffer areas.

☆ Cover freshly added manure in storage pile with stall waste, straw, or old hay to prevent surface exposure of the manure. Prior to addition of fresh manure, the manure pile top should be made flat.

☆ When removing manure from the storage area, leave at least a 4-inch dry pad of old manure/bedding on the bottom of the storage area to provide a stock of beneficial microbes/parasites and decomposer organisms. This will also help to absorb moisture as and when new manure is added.

For many livestock farms, equipments for manure removal are; pitchforks or manure forks, shovels, metal rakes with close tins or even brooms and dust pans, and wheelbarrow or handcart/tractor trolley. A pick-up truck can also be useful.

Manure should be handled carefully to prevent exposure to potential bacteria and protozoa that may be present in it. Sanitary measures, including hand washing before touching food, eyes, *etc.*, or wearing of masks should be strictly followed.

The utilization of manure can be on-farm or off-farm depending upon the land availability. Farms with readily available land can well benefit from land application of manure, however, farms with less land or more manure may need to consider off-farm utilization options or composting. Land application of manure is a low cost option for farmers who have sufficient land space available. Stockpiled manure usually can be applied to the pasture or crop lands at the rate of 10- 40 tons per acre as per the status of soil. Proper land application of manure necessitates to have knowledge of nutrient needs of your soil, the nutrient content of the manure you are applying, and fertilizer needs of the crop or pasture grass you intend to grow. In order to get best nutrient benefits from the manure, apply it as close as possible to planting time. If the nutrient loss is not a concern, apply it in the fall and plant cover crops on it, such as rye or oats. Manure should be harrowed or incorporated into the soil with a rake or tiller within 72 hours of application to reduce the nutrient loss and run-off contamination. Almost all of the total phosphorus and potassium from manure application are available in the first growing season. Nitrogen availability is slower with only about one-third available to crops during the year it is applied, and the remaining becoming available at a rate of about 5 percent a year.

Composting

The manure may be hauled to a compost operation to have the best use of the manure.

Stockpiling or storing of the manure is not composting. Manure that is being stockpiled decomposes very slowly, reduces in volume relatively little, and still maintains the same bacteria and weed seed issues as raw manure. Composting involves the proper mixture of materials, temperature, oxygen, moisture and maintenance of an environment for microbial activity. The microbes or beneficial bacteria and other organisms digest and process the manure and bedding and stabilize the organic material. The process produces heat that, in turn, produces a final product that is stable, free of pathogens, parasites, viable plant seeds and odours and can be beneficially applied to the land. However, composting causes a significant reduction in the nitrogen content of the manure, in particular, of the more readily available inorganic nitrogen fraction.

Composting is receiving increased attention as an alternative manure management practice due to following advantages;

☆ Reduces mass, volume and odour.

☆ Pathogens, parasites and weed seeds are destroyed.

☆ Lowers hauling cost and improves transportability.

☆ Produces soil conditioner, improves nutrient quality and decreases pollutants of soil.

☆ Composting converts the nutrients in manure to stable forms that have a low ability to be lost by volatilization and leaching when applied to the land.

☆ Increases water retention of soil.

☆ Produces saleable product that can be land applied as and when convenient.

However, during composting, there is loss of ammonia, involvement of land, time and labour. Composting may contribute to the greenhouse effect through emission of greenhouse gases.

Under controlled conditions, composting is accomplished in two main stages:

i. Active stage and

ii. Curing stage

In the active composting stage, microorganisms consume oxygen while feeding on organic matter in manure and produces heat, carbon dioxide and water vapour. During this stage, most of the degradable organic matter is decomposed. A management plan is needed to maintain proper temperature, oxygen and moisture for the organisms which can be achieved by turning, aeration and water sprinkling. The highest rates of decomposition occur when temperatures are in the range of 43 - 66°C. During the active composting stage, the temperature may start to fall because of a lack of oxygen, however, turning the material introduces new oxygen and the active composting stage continues. Turning also helps to keep the temperature from reaching the damaging levels. Heat loss can also occur if the pile is too small or is exposed to cold weather. The temperature should be maintained at 55°C or higher for a minimum of 14 days to destroy the viability of many pathogens and weed seeds in the manure.

In the curing phase, microbial activity slows down and as the process nears completion, the material approaches air temperature. Compost is "finished" once all of the available nutrients are used up and the bacterial activity has declined in the pile. When decomposition has been complete or near to complete the temperature in the pile decreases and does not increase even after turning or aeration. Finished compost takes on many of the characteristics of humus, gets reduced in volume, moisture and weight by 20 to 60 per cent, 40 per cent and 50 per cent respectively.

The carbon to nitrogen ratio (C:N) of manure is a very important factor that affects the whole composting process because microbes need 20 to 25 times more carbon than nitrogen to remain active. The ratio should be between 25:1 and 30:1 at the beginning. The microorganisms digest carbon as an energy source and ingest nitrogen for protein and reproduction. Softwood shavings, sawdust and straw are good sources of carbon. If the ratio is too high (insufficient nitrogen), the decomposition slows and if the ratio is too low (too much nitrogen), it is lost to the atmosphere in the form of ammonia.

The minimum desirable oxygen concentration in the composting material is 5 per cent. Greater than 10 per cent is ideal to avoid anaerobic conditions and high odour potential. Rapid aerobic decomposition can only occur in the presence of sufficient oxygen. Aeration occurs naturally when air in the compost gets warmed and rises through the material, that results in drawing-in fresh air from the surroundings at the base of the windrow. Regular mixing of the material or turning enhances aeration in the composting material. Good aeration during composting will encourage complete decomposition of carbon to carbon dioxide, rather than methane.

Moisture plays an essential role in the metabolism of microorganisms and indirectly in the supply of oxygen. Microorganisms can utilize only those organic molecules that are dissolved in water. Moisture content between 50 and 60 per cent (by weight) provides adequate moisture without limiting aeration. If the moisture content falls below 40 per cent, bacterial activity will slow down and will cease entirely below 15 per cent. When the moisture content exceeds 60 per cent, nutrients are leached, porosity is reduced, odours are produced and decomposition slows. Pile tops should be made flat or concave to absorb as much rainfall, snowmelt, or watering as possible. Adequate levels of phosphorus, potassium, carbon, nitrogen *etc.* are important in the composting process and are normally present in the manure. However, during the composting process substantial amounts of nitrogen get lost through ammonia volatilization.

Typically, the composting process will not occur in colder weather. Covering the pile with black plastic will help the pile heat up faster on warmer days. Once weather warms up sufficiently the pile should be turned.

Composting is achieved by following methods:

a. Bin composting is produced by natural aeration and through turning, using a tractor front-end loader. This option is primarily used for composting mortalities, yard waste and smaller amounts of manure.

b. Windrow composting involves piling of raw material in long rows (windrows) and turning at intervals using mobile equipment like tractors with front loaders or compost-turners, machines specially designed for compost turning. This process requires an extensive area. The base of the area can be compacted soil, however, concrete flooring is ideal with the facility to collect any leachate. Windrow composting can either be passive or active.

   i. Passive windrow composting is most common method in which the conventional piles or windrows are aerated through natural ventilation over long periods of time. The compost normally will require years to stabilize. Generally, material to be composted is collected and promptly piled into windrows, which remain untouched. The materials may be wetted before they are initially formed into windrows but this is not essential. Passive aeration has been successfully used in composting manure from dairy cattle and sheep. The center of a windrow quickly becomes anaerobic and by turning, a new supply of oxygen is pumped in.

   ii. Active windrow composting is the production of compost in windrows using mechanical aeration by a front-end loader or a specially designed windrow turner. Turned windrow composting represents a low technology and medium labour approach and produces a uniform product. Windrow composting can produce excellent compost using a variety of diverse materials/wastes such as manure solids and paunch manure (offal).

c. Aerated static pile composting is the production of compost in piles or windrows with mechanical aeration and an air source such as perforated plastic pipes, aeration cones or a perforated floor. Perforated pipes are laid on the floor and covered with porous material like straw, wood chips, *etc.* This stimulates efficient distribution of air. The raw material is then piled on the base and covered with a layer of matured compost to provide thermal insulation and partial odour removal. Aeration, controlled by temperature feedback, is used to sustain the pile in an aerobic state, with proper temperature in the pile and to control the moisture content. Aeration is accomplished either by forcing or drawing air through the compost pile. Aeration systems can be relatively simple using electrical motors, fans and ducting, or they can be more sophisticated incorporating various sensors and alarms.

d. In-vessel composting is the production of compost in drums, silos or channels using a high-rate controlled aeration system designed to provide optimal conditions. It ensures homogeneous composting, inactivation of pathogens and odour reduction. In-vessel composting includes temperature control and is usually a multistage process. Pre-composting or full composting is achieved in the first stage in a bioreactor, and the final composting and maturing in windrows. The most common types of reactors are horizontal and vertical plug-flow and, also, an agitated bin reactor. Some systems incorporate computer control of temperature and oxygen levels. Aeration of the material is accomplished by continuous agitation using aerating machines which operate in concrete bays or by fans providing air flow from ducts built into concrete floors. This type of composting is faster than the previous systems but have more complicated control and processing mechanisms that require costly maintenance which becomes a limiting factor for farmers to opt for this system of composting.

Uses of Compost

☆ Composted manure is safer than the raw manure as a soil amendment.

☆ It is used as a fertilizer supplement, top dressing for pastures and hay crops, mulch for home gardens.

☆ It increases the organic matter and decreases the bulk density or penetration resistance.

☆ It is low in soluble salts, so it will not burn plants.

☆ It can be applied directly to the growing vegetable crops.

☆ It is less likely to cause nutrient imbalances.

☆ It is typically pH-neutral.

☆ It contains less nitrogen than fresh manure; however, nitrogen is more stable and less susceptible to leaching.

☆ It increases the water and nutrient retention of the soil, provides a porous medium for roots to grow.

☆ Compost application rates can typically be as much as 40 to 60 tons per acre on low fertility soils or as little as 10 tons per acre on soils with higher fertility.

☆ It is recommended to spread about ¼ inch of compost on fields three to four times a year.

Vermicomposting

A new concept in efficient management of manure is vermicomposting. Earthworms live in the soil and feed on decaying organic material and transform organic waste to efficient organic, neutral and odourless fertilizer in the shape of worm castings. Vermicomposting is thus a process of turning organic debris into worm castings. The castings are rich in humus and nutrients, contain high amounts of carbon, nitrogen, potassium, phosphorus, calcium, and magnesium. Castings contain, 5 times the available nitrogen, 7 times the available potash, and 1 ½ times more calcium than found in good topsoil. Earthworm castings have excellent aeration, porosity, structure, drainage, and moisture-holding capacity.

Vermicomposting is accomplished in following steps:

1. Collection of Manure along with Bedding Material

The management practices observed in collection and storage of manure has been discussed above in detail.

2. Pre-digestion of Manure

Before worms are engaged in composting the manure, it is necessary to predigest the sheep and goat manure along with beddings like straw, plant residues to decompose the material for action of worms. Pre-digestion is simply achieved by composting the manure along with other organic wastes thermophilically for two months and mechanically turned over every 15 days (refer composting of manure). Sheep and goat manure being relatively dry and pelleted may be mixed with cattle dung slurry and or horse dung and extra bulking material like hay, straw *etc.* during composting.

3. Preparation of Earthworm Bed

it is prerequisite to maintain the worms for composting. For vermicompost production, the surface dwelling earthworm alone should be used. The African earthworm (*Eudrillus engenial*), Red worms (*Eisenia foetida*) and composting worm (*Peronyx excavatus*) are promising worms used for vermicompost production. All the three worms can be mixed together for vermicompost production. Vermiculture bed or worm bed can be prepared by placing saw dust or husk or coir waste or shredded paper combined with typical on-farm organic resources such as straw and hay in the bottom of tub/container (3cm). A layer of fine sand (3 cm) should be spread over the culture bed followed by a layer of garden soil mixed with some aged or composted cattle or sheep manure (3 cm). All layers must be moistened with water. In general, it should be noted that the selection of bedding materials is a key to successful vermiculture or vermicomposting. Bedding is any material that provides the worms with a relatively stable habitat. Worms can be enormously productive (and reproductive) if conditions are good; however, their efficiency drops off rapidly when their basic needs are not met. Good bedding mixtures are an essential element in meeting those needs. Since worms breath through skin, therefore must have moist environment and bedding having ability to absorb and retain water is ideal. The bedding should have good bulking potential, too dense or tightly packed material reduces flow of air thus cannot be a good bedding. The bedding material should have high carbon: nitrogen ratio, as high nitrogen bedding rapidly degrades and produces heat making bedding inhospitable to the worms.

4. Vermicomposting Situates

Compost worms are big eaters. Under ideal conditions, they are able to consume in excess of their body weight each day, although the rule-of-thumb is ½ of their body weight per day. They will eat almost anything organic (that is, of plant or animal origin), but they definitely prefer some foods to others. Manures are the most commonly used worm feedstock, with dairy and beef manures generally considered the best natural food for them. Sheep and goat manure first pre-digested and moisture adjusted to 60 per cent has been successfully used in vermicomposting.

The vermicomposting is carried in containers or compost pits. When the materials available for vermicomposting is limited, it can be proceeded in wooden boxes, plastic buckets, cement tubs. A cement tub may be constructed to a height of 2½ feet and a breadth of 3 feet. The length may be fixed to any level depending upon the size of the room. The bottom of the tub is made to slope like structure to drain the excess water from vermicompost unit. In commercial farms many compost pits can be prepared under a single roof. Compost pits can be dug in an elevated area near the barns to a depth of 2 ½ feet, breadth of 3 feet and length of 10 feet with proper roofing. Bricks or hollow concrete blocks are arranged on all the sides including the floor of the pit to make the pit worm-proof so as to restrict the penetration of worms in the soil.

The pre-digested manure should be mud with 25-30 per cent cattle dung (semidried) either by weight or volume. The mixed waste is placed into the tub/container/pit up to the brim. The moisture level should be maintained at 60 per cent. Over this material, the selected earthworms are placed uniformly. For one-meter square bed 2.5 kg earthworms should be added. There is no necessity that earthworm should be put inside the waste rather they will move inside of its own. It is not necessary to water the compost bed every day, however, 60 per cent moisture should be maintained throughout the period. Water should be sprinkled over the bed rather than pouring the water. During the course of vermicomposting wet gunny bags should be applied on to the top of beds to provide shade as well as reduce desiccation.

5. Collection of Vermicompost

In the tub method of composting, the castings formed on the top layer are collected periodically. The collection may be carried out once in a week. With hand the casting will be scooped out and put in a shady place as a heap. The harvesting of casting should be limited up to earthworm presence on top layer. This periodical harvesting is necessary for free air flow and retain the compost quality. Otherwise the finished compost gets compacted when watering is done. In bed type of vermicomposting method, periodical harvesting is not required. Since the height of the waste material heaped is not much, the produced vermicompost will be harvested after the process is over. It may take some two months for complete vermicomposting and during this period turning of manure and maintenance of moisture should be observed. Watering should be stopped before the harvest of vermicompost.

6. Collection of Earthworms after Vermicomposting

After the vermicompost production, the earthworm present in the tub/small bed may be harvested by trapping method. In this method, before harvesting the compost, small, fresh cow dung balls are made and inserted inside the vermibed in five or six places. After 24 hours, the cow dung balls are removed. All the worms will be adhered into the ball. Putting the cow dung ball in a bucket of water will separate the adhered worms. Worms can also be harvested by sieving the vermicompost through nets. The collected worms will be used for next batch of composting. Worm harvesting is usually carried out in order to sell the worms, rather than to start new worm beds. Expanding the operation can be accomplished by placing a new bedding material in the close proximity of vermicompost with worms or remove a portion of the bed to start a new one and replacing the material with new bedding and feed. Within 24 to 48 hours all worms must have migrated of its own in the new bedding.

7. Storing Vermicompost and its Utilization

The harvested vermicompost should be stored in dark, cool place. It should have minimum 40 per cent moisture. It should not be exposed to sunlight that will lead to loss of moisture and nutrient content. It is advocated that the harvested composted material is openly stored rather than packed in over sac. Packing can be done at the time of selling. If it is stored in open place, periodical sprinkling of water may be done to maintain moisture level and also to maintain beneficial microbial population. However, compost can be stored/packed in laminated, air proof bags that will minimize the evaporative moisture loss. Vermicompost can be stored for one year without loss of its quality, if the moisture is maintained at 40 per cent level. Vermicompost has some below inked qualities that makes it the best soil moderator.

☆ Vermicompost is rich in all essential plant nutrients and is used as a soil improver.

☆ It is rich in beneficial micro flora such as fixers, P- solubilizers, cellulose decomposing micro-flora *etc.* that improve soil environment.

☆ It provides excellent effect on overall plant growth. It improves soil structure, texture, aeration, and water-holding capacity and prevents soil erosion.

☆ It is free flowing, easy to apply, handle and store and does not have bad odour.

☆ It is free from pathogens, toxic elements, weed seeds *etc.* thus a good soil amendment than raw manure.

Chapter 11

Farm Project Report

A scheme can be prepared by a beneficiary for establishing a farm after consulting technical persons of State Sheep Husbandry Departments, Sheep development Boards, commercial farmers, experts in financing institutions and or farming or research institutes. Beneficiaries should also visit progressive farmers and government/agricultural university farm establishments in the vicinity and discuss the profitability of farming with stakeholders. These agencies besides providing full technical support shall also provide all support in marketing of live animals and wool.

While preparing a project, information on land, availability of water, feeds, fodder, veterinary aid, breeding facilities, livestock markets, marketing aspects, training facilities, experience of the farmer and the type of assistance available from State Government, or other agencies should be readily available. The farmer should have knowledge of different breeds of animals to be purchased, their production performance, cost and other relevant input and output costs with their description before starting the farming. Based on this, the total cost of the project, margin money to be provided by the beneficiary, requirement of bank loan, estimated annual expenditure, income, profit and loss statement, repayment period, *etc.* can be worked out and included in the project.

Requirements of a Good Project

NABARD and many other banks are entertaining the schemes for establishment of a sheep/goat farm. The scheme so formulated should be submitted to the nearest branch of bank. The bank's officers can assist in preparation of the scheme or filling in the prescribed application form. The bank will then examine the scheme for its technical feasibility and economic viability.

The general format for the scheme is as under;

Scheme: Sheep/Goat Breeding/Rearing

1. General

    i. Name of the sponsoring bank

    ii. Address of the controlling office sponsoring the scheme

    iii. Nature and objective of the proposed scheme

    iv. Details of proposed investments

    v. Specification of the scheme area (Name of District/Block)

    vi. Names of the financing bank's branches

    vii. Status of beneficiaries: (Individual/Partnership/Company/Corporation/ Co-operative Society/Others)

    viii. In case of area based schemes, coverage of borrowers in weaker sections (*viz.* Landless labourers), small, medium and large farmers as per the norms of financial agency.

2. Technical Aspects

a) Animals

    i. Proposed Breed

    ii. Age of the animal

    iii. Arrangements for vaccination, identification and health certificate

    iv. Insurance

    v. Cost of ram

    vi. Cost of ewes

b) Production parameters

    i. Age at first lambing/kidding: (preferably 12 -18 months)

    ii. Lambing/kidding interval: (one year in case of sheep and 08 months in case of goats)

    iii. Lambing/kidding percentage: (75 per cent in lambing, 125 per cent in kidding minimum)

    iv. Number of lambs/kids produced:

    v. Mortality of adults/lambs: (2-5 per cent in adults and 10 per cent in lambs/ kids)

    vi. Age at which lambs are sold: 8- 12 months

    vii. Body weight of lambs/kids: 15-25 kg/animal

c) Housing

    i. Type of housing: (kacha/Pacca)

    ii. Floor space - adults/lambs: 10 sqft. For adults and 4 sqft. for lambs

    iii. Cost of construction: Civil engineering department rates

    iv. Other civil structures (for commercial units)

d) Equipment Needed

    i. Chaff cutter

    ii. Feeding/watering troughs

    iii. Hay/straw racks

    iv. Shearing/clipping equipment

    v. Vaccinators/drenching machines

    vi. Tagging or tattooing equipment

    vii. Surgical Dressing Kit

e) Comments on technical feasibility

f) Government restrictions, if any

3. Financial Aspects

    i. Name of Investment:

    ii. Size of unit:

    iii. Unit Cost (with component-wise break-up (Rs.)

    iv. Whether approved by state level unit Cost Committee

    v. Down payment/margin/subsidy (indicate source and extent of subsidy)

    vi. Year-wise physical and financial program

    vii. Financial viability (comment on the cash flow projection on a farm model/ unit and enclose the same)

    viii. Lending Terms: (Rate of interest, Grace period, repayment period)

    ix. Nature of security:

    x. Availability of Government guarantee wherever necessary

4. Infrastructural Facilities

    i. Availability of animals (Source, Place of purchase, Distance, Type of arrangements for purchase, Availability in required numbers)

    ii. Grazing Land: (Adequacy, Distance, Duration of grazing, Condition of grazing lands, Cost to be paid/animal

    iii. Feeding: (Type of fodder, Source, Cost/animal year, In case of commercial units, area under fodder crops.

    iv. Breeding Cover: (Source, Place, Distance, Type of services available, Availability of staff, Cost/animal/year)

    v. Marketing: (Source for Animals, Milk, Wool, Place, Distance, Price realized - Animals – culls lambs, Wool (Rs./Kg.), Milk (Rs./liter))

    vi. Other aspects: (Source of technical guidance, Training facilities, Other Government Support)

    vii. Supervision and monitoring arrangements available with the bank.

While preparing a project report for a sheep or goat farm following heads should be considered for its preparation;

    1. Non-recurring investment for sheep and goats
        a. Cost of animals
        b. Cost of housing
        c. Cost of infrastructure
    2. Recurring investment or cash flow for sheep and goat farming.
    3. Economics of Sheep and goat farming –techno-economic parameters
        a. Production Traits
        b. Expenditure norms
        c. Income Norms
        d. Repayment Norms
    4. Economics of Sheep and goat farming – flock projection chart
        a. Opening Stock
        b. Births during the year
        c. Mortality
        d. Sales during the year
        e. Closing stock at the end of the year
    5. Economics of farming - cash flow statement
    6. Economics of farming – repayment schedule

Non-recurring Investment for Sheep and Goats

a. Animal Purchase

Goat purchase cost:

35 Kg. X cost/kg live weight = A (per Doe cost)

45 Kg. X cost/kg live weight = B (per Buck cost)

Sheep purchase cost:

35 kg x cost/kg live weight = a (per Ewe cost)

50 kg x cost/kg live weight = b (per Ram cost)

Investment for 1 goat/sheep unit of 50 females + 02 males

Total cost of 50 Does: 50 x A = C

Total cost of 02 Bucks: 02 x B = D

Total cost of 1 unit = G

Or

Total cost of 50 Ewes: 50 x a = c

Total cost of 2 Rams: 02 x b = d

Total cost of 1 unit = S

b. Housing for Sheep and Goats

10 sqft/adult animal and 4 sqft/kid or lamb

For 50 Does/ewes = 50 x 10 sft. = 500 sqft.

For 02 Bucks/rams = 02 x 20 sft. = 40 sqft.

For 70 kids = 70 x 4 sqft. = 280 sqft.

Or

For 50 lambs = 50 x 4 Sqft. =200 sqft

Total = 820 Sqft. for goats and

=740 Sqft. for sheep

c. Infrastructure Cost

Attendant's room (10 x 12) = 120 Sqft @ Rs.

Store room (10 x 20) = 200 Sqft.@ Rs.

Total cost of housing and infrastructure for 1 goat unit = 820 + 120 +200

= 1140 Sqft. X construction cost/Sqft. (X)

Or

Total cost of housing and infrastructure for 1 sheep unit = 740 + 120 + 200

= 1060 sqft. X construction cost/Sqft. (Y)

Total of nonrecurring investment for one unit of sheep or goat (52 animals):

G/S + X/Y= NRC

Recurring Investment

Water, Electricity and other Misc. Expenses

For 1 unit (*i.e.*, 50 Does/ewes and 2 Bucks/rams) is 52 x 20 = Rs.1040/- (approximately Rs. 20/- per animal per year is calculated.

Supplementary Feed Cost

During the summer months there is enough grazing so no need of any supplement but during winter months the animals mostly are stall-fed with hay and concentrate.

Concentrate Feeding Cost

For 50 Does/ewes for 4 months (120 days) = 120 x 50 x 11 = 66,000/(500g/ animal/day @ Rs.22/kg)

For 02 Bucks/rams for 4 months (120 days) = 120 x 02 x 8.8 = 2112/(400g/animal/day @ Rs.22/kg)

Hay Fodder Cost

For 50 Does/ewes for 4 months (120 days) = 120 x 50 x 12 = 72,000/(1.2 kg/animal/day @ Rs.10/kg)

For 02 Bucks/rams for 4 months (120 days) = 120 x 02 x 15 = 3600/(1.5kg/animal/day @Rs. 10/kg)

For 70 Kids for 3 months (90 days) = 90 x 70 x 2.3 = 14490/(creep ration 100g/kid/day @Rs.23/kg)

For 50 lambs for 3 months (90 days) = 90 x 50 x 2.3 = 10350/(creep ration 100g/lamb/day @Rs.23/kg)

Total feed cost of 1 goat unit = 1,58,202/

Total feed cost of 1 sheep unit = 1,54,062/

Insurance

4 per cent of purchase cost of Goats = G x 4 per cent (M)

4 per cent of purchase cost of sheep = S x 4 per cent (N)

Medical and Vet Charges

Per Goat/Ewe = Rs.25/-

For 1 unit of goat or sheep with 52 animal heads = 52 x 25 = Rs.1300/-

Labour Wages

For 1 labourer 12,000 x 12 = 1,44,000/- (per Annum)

Rs. 400/= per day per labourer

Other Instruments

Cost of Feeding Tubs and Iron railing *etc.*, = Rs. 5,000/-

Cost of other equipments/kits = Rs. 4000/-

Total = Rs. 9,000/-

Total of recurring investment:

= Rs. 1040 + 1,58,202/1,54,062 + M/N + 1300 + 144000 + 9000 = RC

Grand total of all the above mentioned items = NRC + RC = GT

Margin Money @ 20 per cent of total cost = GT x 20 per cent = MM

Bank Loan @ 80 per cent of total cost = GT x 80 per cent = BL

Economics of Goat Farming – Techno-Economic Parameters

Income Norms

    i. Sale price of buckling/Ram lamb = (value/kg live weight x body weight)

   ii. Sale price of Doelings/Ewe lamb = (value/kg live weight x body weight)

   iii. Sale of Adult Does/Ewes = (value/kg live weight x doe/ewe weight)

   iv. Sale of Adult Bucks/Rams = (value/kg live weight x buck/ram weight)

   v. Income from manure is not assumed as it is used on the own farm

   vi. Sale of gunny bags = (20 bags/tone x cost of a bag)

   vii. Sale of milk in case of goats = (milk in kg x cost/kg)

   viii. Sale of wool in case of sheep farming = wool produced/animal x No. of animals x Cost per kg wool

Repayment Norms

   i. Repayment period (years) (including grace period) =

   ii. Grace period (years) = 2

   iii. Interest (per cent) = 12 per cent

Economics of Sheep and Goat Farming

A. Flock Projection Chart

Particulars	Years									
	1	2	3	4	5	6	7	8	9	10
Opening stock of Does/ewes	50	48	44	45	37	44	45	37	44	45
Replaced stock	0	02	06	05	13	06	05	13	06	05
Opening stock of Bucks/rams	2	2	2	2	2	2	2	2	2	2
Births during the year										
Male kids/lambs	0	35/25	35/25	35/25	35/25	35/25	35/25	35/25	35/25	35/25
Female kids/lambs	0	35/25	35/25	35/25	35/25	35/25	35/25	35/25	35/25	35/25
Mortality (2-5 per cent adults)	0	01	02	01	–	02	01	–	02	01
Mortality (10 per cent kids/lambs	0	3/2	4/2	3/3	3/2	4/2	3/3	3/2	4/2	3/3
Sale during the year										
Bucks/ram	0	0	0	01	01	0	0	01	01	0
Does/ewes	0	12	12	25	12	12	25	12	12	25
Bucklings/Male hogget	0	0	30/21	30/20	31/21	29/21	31/21	31/22	28/20	31/21
Doelings/Female hogget	0	0	23/15	25/15	18/09	23/15	26/16	18/09	22/14	26/16

B. Costs

   a) Capital cost:

   b) Purchase of livestock:

   c) Feed cost:

     i) Grazing

     ii) Concentrate

    iii) Hay fodder

d) Insurance cost:

e) Veterinary aid:

f) Labour cost:

g) Shearing charges: Rs. 20/sheep x 2 if shearing twice a year

   Total cost:

C. Benefits

a) Sale of young animals:

b) Sale of culled animals:

c) Sale of Wool: (in case of sheep only)

d) Sale of milk: (in case of goats only)

e) Closing stock value:

   Total benefits:

   Net Benefit:

Chapter 12

Determination of Age of an Animal

The age of an animal is an important factor governing its market value. It can be estimated in goats and sheep by looking at the teeth.

Both sheep and goats have a total of 32 teeth. They do not have any upper incisors. The dental formula for sheep and goats is; 0/4 incisors, 3/3 pre-molars, 3/3 molars. The first number in each formula represents how many sets of teeth are on the upper jaw; the second number indicates how many sets of teeth are on the lower jaw. All baby sheep and goats are born with deciduous teeth (teeth that will fall out). Deciduous teeth are much smaller than permanent teeth. The deciduous teeth are replaced with permanent teeth as the animal ages and the appearance of permanent teeth in fact predicts the age of an animal. The following table outlines when the permanent teeth will appear or erupt:

Permanent Tooth Eruption in Sheep and Goats

Permanent Tooth	Age at Eruption
Incisor (I_1)	1-1.5 years
Incisor (I_2)	1.5-2 years
Incisor (I_3)	2.5-3 years
Incisor (I_4)	3.5-4 years
Premolars	1.5-2 years
Molar (M_1)	3 months
Molar (M_2)	9-12 months
Molar (M_3)	1.5-2 years

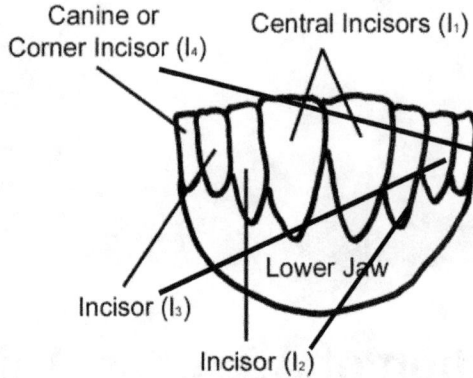

A rough sketch of a set of incisors on lower jaw.

The age of a sheep can be determined by examining the status of permanent set of teeth particularly incisors.

Common Dentition of Sheep

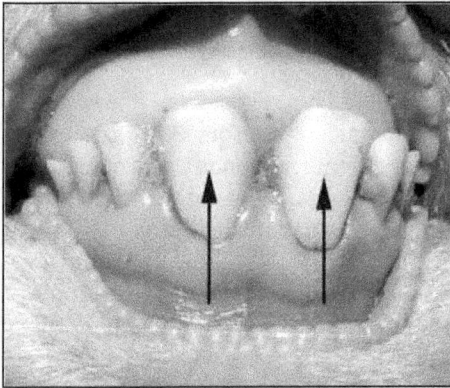

**Dentition of a Yearling Sheep.
Two incisors are permanent.**

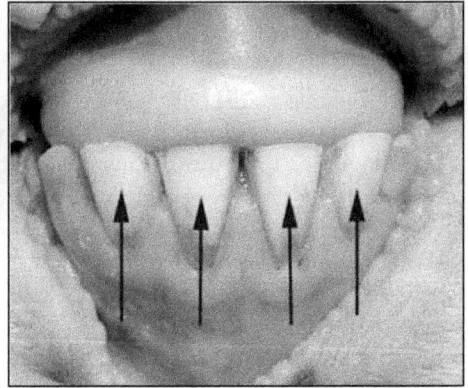

**Dentition of a 2-year-old Sheep.
Four incisors are permanent.**

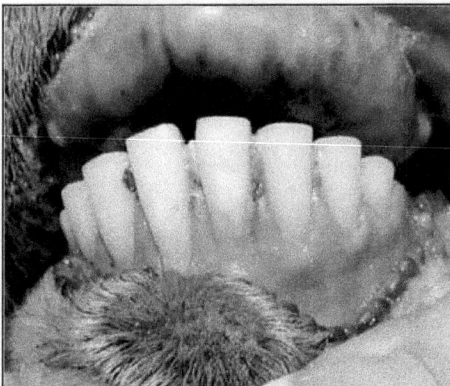

**Dentition of a 4-year-old Sheep or Full
Mouth. All incisors are permanent.**

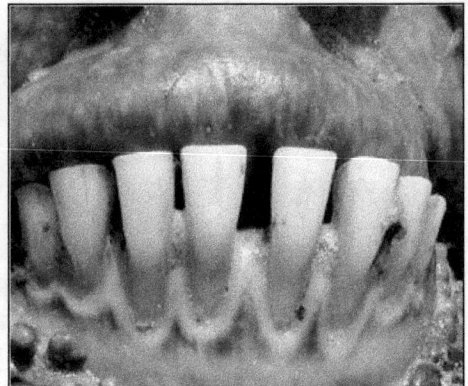

**Dentition of a 6-8-year-old Sheep. Notice
the wide spacing between the teeth.**

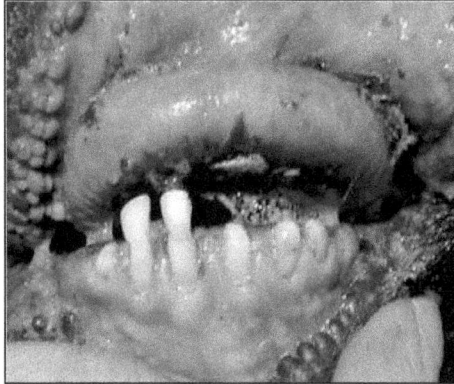

Dentition of an Extremely Aged Sheep (from 8-12 years of age), Frequently Referred to as a "Broken Mouth." Notice how this ewe has severely worn or missing teeth, with receding gum lines.

Common Dentition of Goats

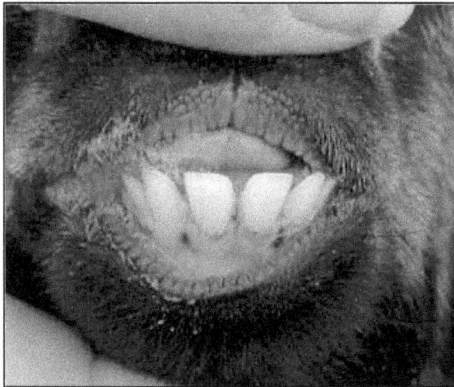

Dentition of a Goat 10 Months of Age. All the teeth are still baby teeth.

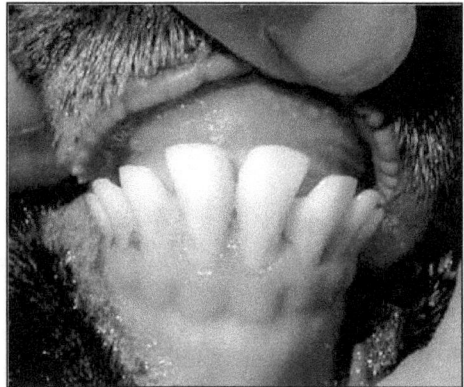

Dentation of a Yearling. Two incisors are permanent.

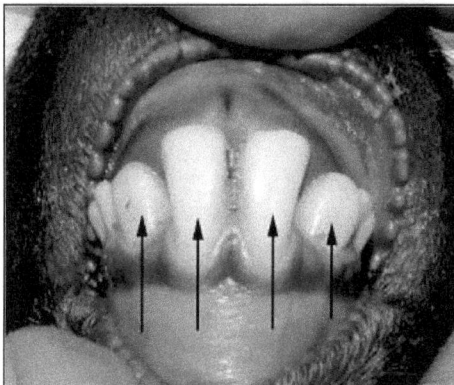

Dentition at 1.5-2 Years Old Goat. Four incisors are permanent.

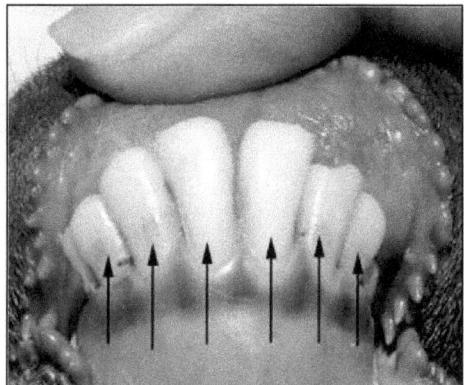

Dentition of a 3-year-old Goat. Six incisors are permanent.

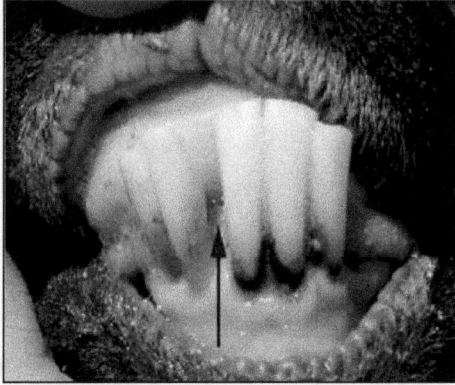

Dentition of an Aged Goat (about 10 years old). All the incisors are permanent and worn. The black arrow shows missing an incisor.

Chapter 13

Interesting Behaviours of Sheep and Goat

Sheep (Ovis aries)	Goat (Capra hircus)
Sheep has a lifespan of 10-12 years	Goat has a life span of 15 – 18 years
Sheep have 54 chromosomes	Goats have 60 chromosomes
Sheep were domesticated 10,000 years ago in Central Asia.	Goat have been found in 10,000-year-old settlement of GanjDerah, in the Near East.
Contrary to popular misconception, sheep are extremely intelligent animals capable of problem solving. They are considered to have a similar IQ level to cattle and are nearly as clever as pigs.	Goats are very intelligent and curious animals. Their inquisitive nature is exemplified in their constant desire to explore and investigate anything unfamiliar which they come across.
Like various other species including humans, sheep make different vocalizations to communicate different emotions. They also display and recognize emotion by facial expressions.	Goats communicate with each other by bleating. Mothers will often call to their young (kids) to ensure they stay close-by.
Sheep are highly social and closely related and always remain in flocks. "Get one to go and they will all go."	Goats are social animals, however unlike sheep, they are not flock-orientated. They are tolerant of interaction in general.

Sheep (Ovis aries)	Goat (Capra hircus)
Female sheep (ewes) are very caring mothers and form deep bonds with their lambs that can recognize them by their call (bleat) when they wander too far away.	Mother and kid goats recognize each other's calls soon after the mothers give birth. Kids are very close to their mothers.
Sheep have an upper lip that is divided by a distinct philtrum (groove).	Goats do not have groove in their lips.
Sheep are grazers, preferring to eat short, tender grasses and clover. Their dietary preference is forbs (broadleaf weeds) and they like to graze close to the soil surface.	Goats are natural browsers, preferring to eat leaves, twigs, vines, and shrubs. They are very agile and will stand on their hind legs to reach vegetation. Goats like to eat the tops of plants.
Sheep have better resistance to pasture parasites because of being close grazers. The clostridial vaccines also seem to be more effective in sheep than goats.	Goats are less resistant to pasture parasites because they eat off the ground and seldom have contact with parasites on the ground. Goats also metabolize anthelmintics quicker and require higher doses of the drugs.
Sheep are sure footed animals and graze high land pastures. They are close grazers prefer to nibble shorter grasses but will also select flower heads.	They have great balance and are thus able to survive in precarious areas such as steep mountains. They can even climb trees and some species can jump over 5 feet high.
Sheep have a hanging tail	Goats frequently held tail up unless it is sick or frightened
Sheep grows wool.	Goats grow hair.
Ram (male sheep), when aggressive, will butt head-on	Bucks (male goats) will rear up and come down with their heads
Sheep remain without shelter mostly.	Goats will seek shelter more readily than sheep.
Prefer upland grazing to lowland, do not like to get its feet wet.	Also prefer upland grazing to lowland. Again do not like its feet to get wet.
Sheep have face or tear glands beneath their eyes and foot or scent glands between the toes.	Male goats have glands beneath their tail. Male goats develop a distinct odor as they grow in sexual maturity.
Many breeds of sheep are naturally hornless (polled). Some sheep have manes. Sheep tend to curl their horns in loops on the sides of their heads	Most goats are naturally horned. Some goats have beards. Goat horns are more narrow, upright, and less curved
The estrous (heat) cycle of the ewe averages 17 days	The doe's estrous cycle averages 21 days.
Ewes have a more complicated cervix which makes artificial insemination very difficult.	Goats are much easier to artificially inseminate.
Sheep show few visible signs of estrus as compared to goats	Goats have some clear signs of estrus, like swollen vulva, flicking of tail, restlessness, mucous discharge etc.
Sheep are seasonal breeders and mostly bear singles.	Goats tend to be less seasonal and more prolific than sheep.

Sheep (Ovis aries)	Goat (Capra hircus)
Sheep convert feed more efficiently. Grain-feeding is more profitable in mutton production.	Goats have higher maintenance requirements. Grain-feeding is less likely to be profitable in goat production.
Sheep deposit external fat before depositing internal fat.	Goats deposit fat around their internal organs before depositing external fat over their back, ribs, and loin.
Sheep have a narrow tolerance for excess copper in their diet, however there is a breed variation in copper toxicity.	Goats require more copper in their diets than sheep and are not as sensitive to copper toxicity. Can be fed grain and mineral mixtures formulated for other livestock.
OPP (ovine progressive pneumonia) in sheep caused by a slow virus.	CAE (caprine arthritic encephalitis) in goats caused by same slow virus like HIV.
Rams will dominate when kept with bucks, because the ram will preemptively strike the buck in the abdomen while the buck is still in the act of rearing up.	Goats will usually dominate sheep, especially if they have horns. Goats are used as leaders in sheep flocks.
Sheep in the Chinese zodiac are seen to represent righteousness, sincerity, gentleness, and compassion.	The goat in the Chinese zodiac represents introversion, creativity, shyness and being a perfectionist.
Sheep were smuggled into the States during the 16th and 17 centuries to develop the wool industry. Wool is durable, insulating, wrinkle-resisting, and moisture-absorbing and an ideal fabric for sweaters, coats, rugs, blankets and much more.	Goats discovered coffee! Apparently in Ethiopia a goat herd saw goats behaving more actively and energetically after eating from a particular bush. He then tried it himself and felt uplifted, awake and full of energy.
President Woodrow Wilson grazed sheep on the White House lawn.	Abraham Lincoln's sons had two goats that lived in the white house with them.
The ancient Sumerians (4000 – 2000 BCE), who are thought to have developed the first form of writing (Cuneiform script), immortalized sheep in the form of gods in their religion.	The latin 'Capra' is the root of the word 'capricious' which means quirky, whimsical, fanciful and apt to change suddenly.
In 1996 "Dolly", a Finnish Dorset Sheep was the first mammal to be cloned from an adult cell.	In 2012 "Noori" was first Pashmina goat cloned from an adult somatic cell.
Sheep's eye is rectangular rather than round. They have excellent night vision.	Goats too have rectangular eyes and will often browse during the night.
The meat of sheep is widely eaten by people across the world.	Mahatma Gandhi consumed goat milk every day for more than 30 years.

Common Terms Used in Sheep and Goats

Particulars	Sheep	Goats
Adult Male	Ram/Tup	Buck
Adult Female	Ewe	Doe
New born	Lamb	kid
Young male	Ram lamb/Tup lamb	Buckling
Young female	Ewe lamb/Gimmer lamb	Goatling
Castrated male	Wether/Wedder	Wether/castrated goat
Castrated female	Spayed	Spayed
Yearlings	Hogget	Hogget
Female with offspring	Suckling	Suckling
Act of parturition	Lambing	Kidding
Act of mating	Tupping	Serving
Pregnancy	Gestation	Gestation
Sound produced	Bleating	Bleating
Group	Flock/herd/mob	Flock/Band
Species	Called as Ovine	Caprine
Meat	Mutton	Chevon

Chapter 14

Flock Management Annual Calendar

Lambing normally occurs between January and April, with most lambs being born in March. Since the sheep are seasonal breeders, breeding season starts from late August and lamb crop starts from early February. Kidding does not have any synchronization if not observed in the farm as goats are not seasonal breeders. However most often kidding happens in March-April and or September- October. Young one's are usually pastured with their dams throughout the summer months before being marketed at about five to six months of age. Spring-lambing is more profitable because of having natural reproductive efficiency in spring-lambing and takes advantage of lustre pasture during spring and summer thus reducing exchequer on labour, facilities and purchase of feeds.

The whole year calendar for sheep management can be divided into three major phases which further can be divided into various phases for easy understanding and effective management.

    a. Pre-Lambing (August- January)
       i. Pre-breeding (August)
      ii. Breeding (September – October)
     iii. Post –breeding/Pregnancy (November – early February)
    b. Lambing (February – Early April)
    c. Post Lambing (April –July)
       i. Pre-weaning/Lactation (April – June)
      ii. Post-weaning (June – July)

August (Pre-breeding)

☆ Get the best sheep flock ready for breeding.

☆ Do Breeding Soundness Examination (BSE) on rams and ewes like physical examination of udders and feet of ewes, scrotums and penises of rams, evaluation of semen characteristics if possible, previous history of any infection, abortion or breeding problem.

☆ Cull ewes and rams that are not going to be used for breeding. Aged ewes more than 7 years should be culled.

☆ Ewe lambs more than 30 Kg body weight should be selected for replacement stock.

☆ Check Body Condition Score (BCS) and plan extra feeding with concentrate in poor condition ewes and rams while sorting out in groups.

☆ Do Faecal Egg Counts (FEC) and deworm if needed. It is recommended to deworm the animals before breeding to increase lambing percentage.

☆ Do use broad spectrum deworming agents like Nilzan, Zanil, Fenbendazole, Albendazole etc after consultation of a veterinarian.

☆ Treat animals for external parasites either by dipping or by injecting avermectin/duramectin.

☆ Trim feet and run breeding ewes and rams through a zinc-sulfide footbath.

☆ Ensure mineral supplement (including selenium) daily.

☆ Begin selling surplus lambs or those not selected for breeding.

September and October (Breeding)

☆ Turn rams in with ewes after chalking out the mating plan.

☆ In case breeding is in different sheep breeds, turn selected rams in with selected ewes separately preferably in breeding pens during night and graze the ewes and rams separately during the day.

☆ Use one adult ram to 40 ewes or one male hogget to 25 ewes.

☆ Use a marking harness on rams to monitor breeding activity. The crayons should be checked for wear every two days and the colour of crayon changed every 10 days.

☆ Keep rams with ewes for 40 days. During a 40 day breeding, every ewe should have had the opportunity to cycle and be bred twice.

☆ Keep breeding periods of ewe lambs to 35 days so that only the early maturing, most fertile ewe lambs eventually enter the breeding herd.

☆ Remove rams from ewes and ewe lambs after 35 to 45 days.

☆ Rams should be provided nutritious feed and fodder during the mating months.

☆ Continue selling feeder/market lambs.

☆ Shear the animals.

November (Post-breeding/Pregnancy)

☆ Do FEC and deworm if necessary.

☆ Conduct pregnancy diagnosis, and cull open ewes and ewe lambs.

☆ Introduce concentrate ration in the flock initially@150 gm/ewe/day and gradually increase it to the maximum of 700 gm/ewe/day near to parturition.

☆ Male flock should be maintained on concentrate @ 400 gm/animal/day.

☆ Graze the animals if permitted by weather conditions or use good hay @ 1- 1.5 kg/animal/day.

December and January (Post-breeding/Pregnancy)

☆ Stall fed the livestock.

☆ Provide concentrate @ 500g/ewe/day and good quality hay @ 1-1.5 Kg/ewe/day.

☆ Vaccinate ewes with ETV (Clostridium perfringens type C and D) and tetanus one month before expected lambing.

☆ Add a coccidiostat to the ewes' ration 30 days prior to lambing if needed.

☆ Provide optimum feed and fodder to the ewes.

☆ Prepare lambing jugs and lambing kits (Tincture iodine 5-7 per cent, gloves. Scissors, drapes, lubricants, intrauterine lavages and boluses).

☆ Divide ewes into single and multiple bearing groups and also group separately the ewes with poor body condition and adjust nutrition programs accordingly.

☆ Check the blood glucose level and ketone bodies in the blood regularly and accordingly adjust the ration in the flock.

February/March (Lambing)

☆ Take extra care for nutrition. Provide concentrate 700 g/ewe/day in advanced as well as lactating ewes. Also use molasses in lukewarm drinking water @ 50-100 ml/ewe/day.

☆ Check the blood glucose and ketone body levels in the blood regularly and accordingly adjust the ration in the flock.

☆ Regularly observe ewes for lambing. Keep vigil during night also.

☆ Move the ewes and lambs to lambing jugs after lambing. Lambing jugs provide privacy for the ewe and lambs to bond.

☆ When lambs are born, allow mother to lick it and also assist lambs in suckling the mother. Dry the lambs with dry and clean drapes.

☆ Strip the teats of the ewe to remove the wax plug from the teat canal, and ensure lambs get their first sip of colostrum.

☆ Ensure colostrum feeding of the newborns.

☆ Clip the navel to 1- to 1.5-inch length and dip in 7 per cent tincture of iodine.

☆ Keep jugs warm with use of heaters or infra-red bulbs and have soft and clean bedding in the jugs.

☆ Check lambs and ewes in jugs several times each day to ensure ewes are claiming lambs and lambs are getting enough to eat.

☆ Remove ewes and lambs from jugs after two to three days and place in small group of four to eight ewes with their lambs for further observation. Later combine these groups into a workable size unit.

☆ Ewes with twins should be separated from those with singles. Extra care should be taken for twin lambs and ensure their udder feeding.

☆ Give lambs vitamin E/selenium injections.

☆ Observe lambs for scours, pneumonia, or other problems. Start treatment for scours immediately after sighting problem.

March/April (Lambing)

☆ Start creep-feeding in lambs (30 days of age). Creep feed includes crushed grains and cakes along with mineral mixture.

☆ Dock all lambs and castrate all ram lambs born during the previous week if not used for breeding purpose.

☆ Vaccinate lambs with ETV (multi-component) at an age of one month.

☆ Give anti-coccidial to lambs if needed at 3-4 weeks of age for 5 days and repeat it after 3 weeks.

☆ Screen the lambs for Entropion and Rectal-ani and get the conditions corrected by a veterinarian. Many a times in lambs there is impaction or occlusion or infection of interdigital oil/scent gland that results into limping and can be corrected by applying pressure on the gland pouch which releases the contents or if infected use local as well as systemic antibiotics with the consultation of veterinarian.

☆ Take the flock for grazing if weather permits. Do not abruptly stop hay and concentrate feeding.

April/May (Post-lambing)

☆ Dock all lambs and castrate all ram lambs born during the previous week if practised.

☆ Do FEC on ewes and lambs and deworm if needed.

☆ Booster all lambs at approximately of two months with ETV(multi-component) and tetanus.

☆ Stop creep-feeding and put lambs on growing ration.

☆ Keep lambs born in late February, March, April, and May with their dams while grazing in the spring and throughout most of the summer.

☆ Rotating systems be followed that require moving ewes and lambs every 10 to 14 days and using higher stocking rates.

☆ Approximately two days before weaning, limit feed and water to ewes to prepare them for weaning.

☆ Continuously observe ewes for signs of mastitis and lambs for signs of starvation.

☆ After weaning, lambs maybe left on pasture until they are marketed as feeder or slaughter lambs.

June/July (Post-weaning)

☆ Do FEC and deworm if needed.

☆ Cull ewes that are not going to be bred next year.

☆ Continue to observe ewes for signs of mastitis and lambs for signs of starvation.

☆ Shear ewes and rams. Shearing minimizes heat stress and enhances performance.

☆ Give pre-breeding vaccinations to ewes and replacement ewe lambs as per the vaccination schedule.

☆ Do body condition score and supplement the poor ones.

☆ Place replacement ewe lambs on replacement ration.

☆ Purchase replacement ewes and rams if needed.

☆ Migrate flock to high land pastures in Bhaks if tradition.

Note:

☆ *Yet the above calendar may not be true with goats as long as periods are concerned but there remains no difference in management practices between goats and ewes thus the same calendar will be followed in goats also.*

☆ *Shearing, dipping and deworming preferably twice a year in Spring and Autumn season may be followed.*

☆ *Deworming 2 weeks before vaccination is recommended.*

Vaccination Schedule for Sheep and Goat

Sl.No.	Disease	First Shot	Booster Shot	Repeat Vaccination
1.	Peste-des-Petitis Ruminants (PPR)	3 months of age	Not required	Every 3 years
2.	Foot and Mouth Disease (FMD)	3-4 months of age	3-4 weeks after 1st Injection	Every 6 and 12 month interval
3.	Sheep/Goat Pox (GP)	3-4 month of age	3-4 weeks after 1st Injection	Every 12 month interval
4.	Enterotoxaemia (ETV)	1-3 months of age	3-4 weeks after 1st Injection	Every 6 and 12 month interval
5.	Haemorrhagic Septicaemia (HS)	3-4 months of age	3-4 weeks after 1st Injection	Every 6 and 12 month interval

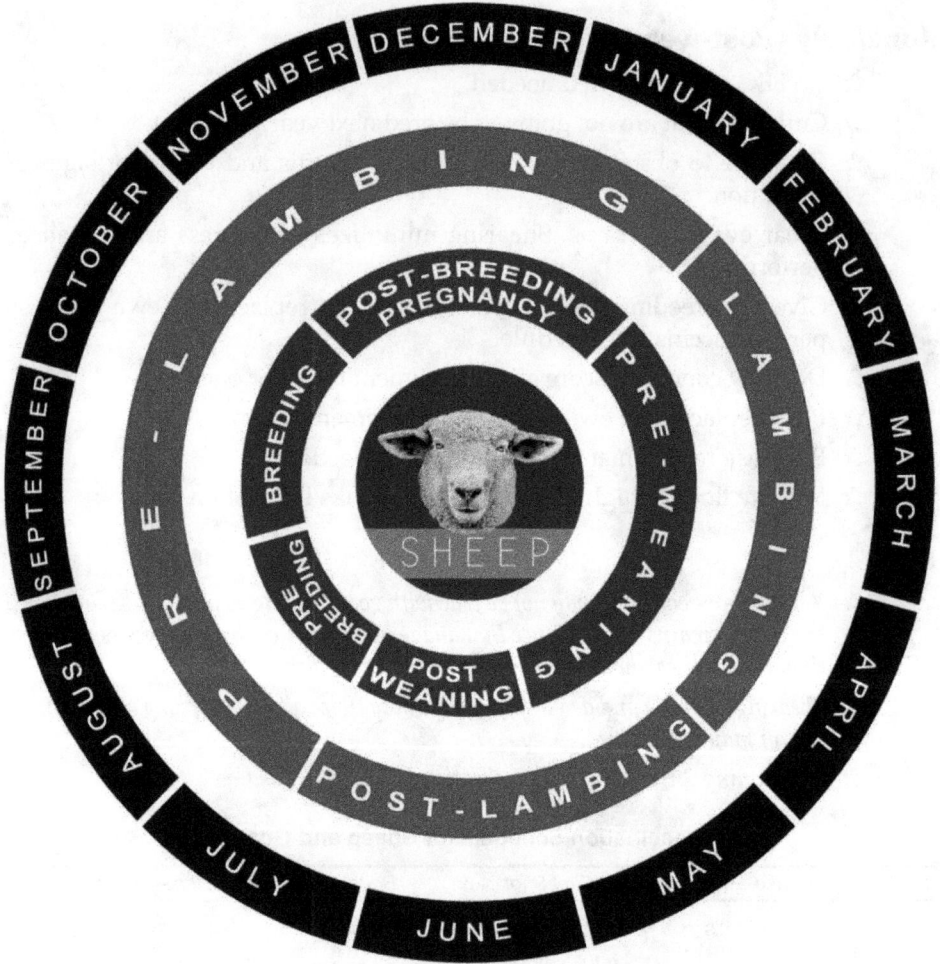

Sheep Management Annual Calendar.

Chapter 15

Physiological Profiles of Sheep and Goats

Important Reproductive Parameters in Female Sheep and Goat

Parameter	Ewe	Doe (goat)
Length of estrous cycle (days)	17	20
Length of estrous	29 hr.	40 hr.
Time of ovulation	Near end of estrous	33 hr after start of estrous
Fertilized ova enter uterus (days)	4 post-estrous	4 post-estrous
Implantation begins at (days)	15 post estrous	20 post estrous
Length of pregnancy(days)	148	148
Type of placenta	Syndes-mo-chorial	Syndes-mo-chorial
Puberty age (months)	6-12	6-12

Important Semen Characteristics in Sheep and Goats

Characteristic Component	Ram	Buck
Ejaculate volume (ml)	0.8-1.2	0.9- 1.5
Sperm concentration (million/ml)	2000-3000	2500-3100
Sperm/ejaculate (billion)	1.6-3.6	2.5 – 3.6
Sperm head(μ)Length/width	8.2/4.25	
Middle pieceLength/width	14/0.80	
Tail pieceLength/width	40-45/0.50	
Motile sperm (per cent)	60-80	70 - 80
Morphologically normal sperm per cent	80-95	82 - 90
Protein (gm/100ml)	5.0	5-6
pH	5.9-7.3	6 – 7.3

Important Haemato-biochemical Profiles of Sheep and Goats

Parameter	Sheep	Goat
Hb (g per cent)	8–16 (12)	8–14 (11)
PCV (per cent)	26–36 (30)	24–36 (30)
RBC (10^6/cumm)	5–11 (8)	10–18 (13)
Diameter of RBC (µ)	4.8	4
RBC surface area (sq.m/kg b.wt.)	58	56
MCV (cu µ)	35	19
MCH (pg)	13	7
MCHC (per cent)	35	35
WBC (10^3/cumm)	4–10 (8)	4–13 (8)
Neutrophils (per cent)	10–50 (30)	30–40 (36)
Lymphocytes (per cent)	50–75 (62)	50–70 (56)
Monocytes (per cent)	0–6 (2.5)	0–4 (2.5)
Eosinophils (per cent)	0–10 (5)	1–8 (5)
Basophils (per cent)	0–3 (0.5)	0–1 (0.5)
Platelets (10^6/cumm)	0.25–0.75	0.2–0.5
ESR(mm)	00/hr.	00/hr.
Heart rate (beats/min)	70–80	70–80
Blood volume (ml/kg)	58–74	70
Plasma volume (ml/kg)	46–53	53
Mean blood pressure (mm Hg)	110	120
CardiacOut put (ml/kg/min)	107–114	129
Bleeding time (min)	1–4	1–4
Clotting time (min)	1.5 – 2.5	2.5
Rectal temp.(ºF)	102.3	103.8
Respiration rate (breaths/min)	19	19
Blood glucose (mg per cent)	35–74	45–60
Blood urea nitrogen (mg per cent)	8–20	13–28
Blood uric acid (mg per cent)	0.05–2	0.3–2
Blood Creatinine (mg per cent)	1–2	1–2
Total plasma protein (g per cent)	6–7.9	6.4–7.9
Serum total cholesterol (mg per cent)	100–150	55–200
Serum calcium (mg per cent)	11.4	10.7
Serum phosphorus (mg per cent)	5.1 – 9	3 –11
Bilirubin (mg per cent)	0–0.39	0 – 0.1
Alkaline phosphatase (iu/L)	5 – 30	7 –30
SGOT (iu/L)	68 – 80	43 –132
SGPT (iu/L)	10 – 12	7 –24

Index